"This book is exactly what ev[...]
throes of midlife needs. Mikala [...]
encouraging women in their physical, emotional, and spiritual journeys as they navigate the complexities of this season of their lives. Her wisdom and expertise, along with her gentle and caring heart, leap off the pages of this book. It's a must-read."

Esther Joy Goetz, author, spiritual director, podcast hostess, and creator of Moms of Bigs and The Dolly Mama

"Dr. Albertson delves into the heart of women navigating midlife. She approaches hot topics within the health and wellness community with a warm hug, a guiding hand, and a soothing voice, letting us know we are not alone as we travel this season of life."

Ali Flynn, author and creator of Hang in There, Mama

"If ever there was a book you need to not only read but keep on your bedside table for all the days, this is it. Mikala's deep knowledge of what is happening in our bodies accompanied by her deep knowledge of what is happening in our hearts makes this a must-read for every woman."

Amy Betters-Midtvedt, writer, speaker, educator, and author of *You'll Make It (and They Will Too): Everything No One Talks About When You're Parenting Teens*

"I have watched too many women suffer in silence through these middle years, and I refuse to walk that path. Thank you, Mikala, for paving the way. This book is exactly what we need."

Leslie Means, founder of Her View From Home and bestselling author of *So God Made a Mother*

"As a therapist working primarily with women in their midlife, every word of this book feels like it is speaking directly to so many of my clients. Not only do Mikala's words provide valuable knowledge, they also will leave women in their midlife feeling seen, understood, and valued."

Jenni Brennan, therapist, author, and creator of Changing Perspectives with Jenni Brennan

EVERYTHING
I WISH I COULD
TELL YOU
ABOUT MIDLIFE

Books By Mikala Albertson, MD

Ordinary on Purpose
Everything I Wish I Could Tell You about Midlife

EVERYTHING I WISH I COULD * TELL YOU * ABOUT MIDLIFE

A WOMAN'S GUIDE TO HEALTH IN THE BODY YOU *ACTUALLY* HAVE

MIKALA ALBERTSON, MD

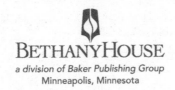

BETHANYHOUSE

a division of Baker Publishing Group

Minneapolis, Minnesota

© 2024 by Mikala Albertson

Published by Bethany House Publishers
Minneapolis, Minnesota
BethanyHouse.com

Bethany House Publishers is a division of
Baker Publishing Group, Grand Rapids, Michigan

Printed in the United States of America

Library of Congress Cataloging-in-Publication Data
Names: Albertson, Mikala, author.
Title: Everything I wish I could tell you about midlife : a woman's guide to health in the body you actually have / Mikala Albertson.
Description: Minneapolis, Minnesota : Bethany House, a division of Baker Publishing Group, [2024] | Includes bibliographical references.
Identifiers: LCCN 2024000774 | ISBN 9780764242984 (paperback) | ISBN 9780764243899 (casebound) | ISBN 9781493447985 (ebook)
Subjects: LCSH: Middle-aged women--Health and hygiene. | Middle-age--Health aspects.
Classification: LCC RA778 .A4367 2024 | DDC 613/.04244--dc23/eng/20240324
LC record available at https://lccn.loc.gov/2024000774

The examples in this book are composites based on the author's experience talking and corresponding with hundreds of patients and website visitors over many years. All names are invented, and any resemblance between these accounts and actual persons is coincidental.

Cover design by Faceout Studio, Spencer Fuller

The Author is represented by The Blythe Daniel Agency, Inc.

Baker Publishing Group publications use paper produced from sustainable forestry practices and postconsumer waste whenever possible.

24 25 26 27 28 29 30   7 6 5 4 3 2 1

For Lizzy,
The woman I am blessed to raise.

My darling, sometimes I wish you could know all the things I've learned the hard way so you would never have to feel pain. Or sadness. Or even an ounce of shame. But I suppose if you did already know, you might miss the incredible, breathtaking beauty of actually *living a life*. Full of trials and hardships and missteps and real Truth and wonderful, ordinary JOY.

As it is, I will be content to walk alongside you, loving you as you go and offering support whenever you need me. I love you, sweetheart.

And I love being your mom.

CONTENTS

DISCLAIMERS

A few stories in this book discuss sensitive topics that may be triggering, including body dysmorphia and eating disorders, substance use, grief, suicidal ideation, abuse, cutting, and trauma. As you come upon a topic you feel could be a personal trigger, please be encouraged to skip those sections or entire chapters if it feels most comfortable for you.

The stories in this book are mine or have been adapted from real events told to me by patients, friends, neighbors, or acquaintances. Whenever necessary, the names, identifying details, and some surrounding circumstances have been changed to maintain the anonymity of all individuals involved.

This is a book for women. Throughout this book, I use the terms *woman* and *women* to describe genetic females. However, I recognize that not all people born with genetically female chromosomes identify as female and vice versa. I encourage you to consider transgender and gender nonbinary individuals as part of the larger group discussed here.

Please also remember that each human being is unique. I am a white, upper-middle class, heterosexual, able-bodied, and educated woman. And while I've worked to learn from and incorporate a wide variety of perspectives here, I want to acknowledge my privilege. I recognize that many women face significant discrimination and resultant barriers to health particularly around race, ethnicity, socioeconomic status, gender and sexuality, ability, and size. Though I've attempted to present the data in a universal way for women *in general*, all of it may not apply to you and your very specific parameters. Your team of personal healthcare providers will always be the best source of information for questions, concerns, and treatments related specifically to YOU.

The scientific principles presented in this book are based upon sound clinical research and backed by a plethora of current articles and books within the citations section. The recommendations and information provided here are up to date as of spring 2024, but it is important to note that science is ever-changing.

Finally, I understand that many readers will have their own ideas and opinions on some of the material presented in this book. So, in the words of the recovery movement, please feel free to "take what you like and leave the rest."

I am honored to have you here.

INTRODUCTION

This is a book for any woman who has reached midlife and wondered, *Is this . . . it? I thought it would get easier. I thought I would have more figured out by now. I always thought life would be more beautiful than this. Something is wrong, and I can't put my finger on it. I'm not the mother or partner I wanted to be. I'm not as successful as I hoped I could be. And, despite the growing pile of self-help books on my bedside table, I'm not turning out to be who I thought I would be. I'm just . . . tired, I guess. Maybe it's my thyroid.*

Which is basically every woman I know, including me.

I've been a family practice doctor for nineteen years. I'm a mom of five children and a wife to a brilliant physician and recovering drug and alcohol addict in recovery now for over fifteen years. I'm a daughter. A sister. A friend. I'm a published author and writer with an online community where each month I may reach millions of women with my words. And every day, I'm trying to figure this life out, too. Still. Just like you. Each day I'm confronted with the truth that this one precious life in my one and only body is harder than I ever imagined it would be, and to be honest, sometimes I feel duped (yes, I've had my thyroid checked multiple times these last few years). I always hoped life would be more beautiful than this, didn't you?

Yeah, me too.

I sent the first proposal for this book to my editor at the beginning of October, a month after my kids started back to school for the year. Our oldest of five children had just begun his senior year in high school and seemed singularly focused on playing basketball, and our youngest child, and only daughter, was off to full-day kindergarten. Suddenly for six hours every day, my house was silent and empty except for our dog, Fern, who regularly hounded me for walks, and our kitten, Tilly, who occasionally peed on any wet towels left scattered on the bathroom floor.

I found myself in one of those new "seasons" people talk about, and the silence of my days was magical. I had many plans for what I might do with this time—exercise classes I would take, closets I hoped to organize, friends I looked forward to catching up with, all the writing I wanted to accomplish. Except occasionally in those first few weeks of silence, I spontaneously burst into tears while loading clothes into the dryer or lying in savasana at the end of yoga. *What was I doing with my one precious, beautiful life?*

I wanted to write about midlife and life transitions (especially career transitions since I left my part-time position with Onsite Care Clinics, where I have worked for the past ten years, and began introducing myself as a "doctor, author, and well-being advocate" in my author bio). I wanted to write about how we are constantly trying to figure out who we are, where we're heading, and what is the meaning of our lives. But my publisher wasn't sold on the idea exactly as it was. So instead, I met mom friends for lunch and walked my dog in endless loops around the path behind our house and finished our family's Christmas shopping long before Thanksgiving week arrived.

In hushed phone conversations with my closest girlfriends, we discussed the calamities of midlife—things like a cheating husband, a teenager forced into nonconsensual sex with a "friend" after a night of partying at college, a tween searching for porn on the iPad, and an aging father who was in and out of the hospital with failing kidneys. We spoke of our looming life doubts and troubled relationships and debilitating fatigue and motherhood angst and horrible periods. Sometimes my friend Angela texted memes of a bloody Carrie from that old Steven King movie to describe her current level of hormonal bleeding. Life seemed . . . hard. And, as the holidays ramped up, I spent most mornings typing at the rickety little Ikea desk perched under the window of my office in our silent home.

Maybe I could write about healing? After all, I've been practicing medicine for nearly two decades, and I had recently renewed my board certification to maintain an active and unrestricted medical license. Plus, since releasing my first book about surrendering perfect, I am attempting to unpack the hurts I've had shoved away for most of my life and rid myself from the shame of childhood sexual abuse hidden under my lengthy list of shiny exterior accomplishments. I go to therapy regularly, and each day I am working on *my own* healing.

The publisher perked up a little at that idea. Yes, maybe there was something there! Healing. That's a topic that might help a wide range of readers. So, I sent off a second proposal for a book about childhood traumas and hurts and the pain we carry into adulthood alongside women's general weariness during midlife and the ongoing process of healing right in this middle part of a hard, messy life. But that wasn't *quite* it either.

I was leaning against the kitchen counter one afternoon, eating directly from a super-sized bag of Ruffles from Costco and scrolling aimlessly on my phone, when the politely worded email from my editor came through:

> Mikala, we love the idea of a book on healing. But I wonder if you could lean into your medical expertise a bit more. Could you write each chapter on topics like the thyroid, depression, insomnia, and

hormones? Perhaps the pitch of the book can be about healing from these very *real* issues women are facing. We're looking for a hopeful message that the best of life is yet to come. And we might want to steer away from any talk of "weariness." Check out this comparable title. The team is excited!

I shoved a few more chips into my mouth and clicked the link. A book with a chiseled middle-aged woman in a sports bra titled *Next Level: Your Guide to Kicking Ass, Feeling Great, and Crushing Goals through Menopause and Beyond* popped up on the screen. It had thousands of five-star reviews.[1]

I thought about Maureen.

When she came to see me as a patient in clinic years ago, it looked like her brown and gray speckled hair hadn't been combed in days. Her eyes were hollow-appearing and rimmed with dark circles underneath. Her hands were trembly. And when I closed the exam room door behind me, she immediately burst into tears and fished a crumpled Kleenex from her purse.

"Oh, Dr. Albertson! I'm sorry. I'm such a mess, look at me. I just need help, and I couldn't find time to shower before I came in. I'm sorry."

I smiled and shook my head at her unnecessary excuses, then shoved my paperwork aside and rolled my little round doctor's stool so close that our knees were nearly touching as the heartbreaking details of a very *real* issue she was facing came tumbling out.

"He's been struggling, and we knew it. We knew! I just hoped we could get him through school, you know? Get him graduated and off to college. I thought maybe he'd meet some friends in college. Some people who would accept him for . . . him."

I listened.

"He's different. We always knew he was different. And kids can be *so* mean. It's my fault. I should've switched him to another school years ago. Or something. I should've done something! We tried counseling and medication. We talked to the principal. But I knew it wasn't helping."

She wiped at the tears spilling down her cheeks and blew her nose with those trembly hands before she went on, "I should've been there."

Her teenage son Jason was admitted to an inpatient hospital room on the psychiatric floor after attempting suicide. He'd been bullied at school for years, and it was all becoming more than he could bear. What could I possibly say? Is there a worse feeling for a mother to endure than watching her child suffer? How could anyone step in and "fix" the helplessness and dread of this situation?

I listened some more. It sounded like Jason was in good hands at the hospital with both a psychiatrist and a therapist he liked. There were individual counseling sessions and group therapy and medication. Plus, a support group for the parents. But Maureen came to see me because she needed help with sleep. She needed something for her trembling hands.

"Honestly, I haven't been feeling well for a while, you know. Mike is semi-retired now, but I'm still working quite a few hours. And not really sleeping. I've been gaining weight. And I'm just . . . tired, I guess. I've been wanting to make an appointment for months to check my thyroid. Because . . ." her voice trailed away. "Dr. Albertson, do you think it could be my thyroid?"

"Maybe. I'm happy to check it."

After a quick exam, I clicked orders into the computer for blood work to rule out causes of fatigue like anemia or hypothyroidism. Then I started her on something for anxiety and gave her an as-needed medication she could use occasionally for sleep. We talked about what self-care looks like during times of crisis—things like scheduled meals and at least weekly therapy and walks around the neighborhood, not for exercise really but just for moving forward. We talked about sleep hygiene and the necessity of rest. We talked about asking for help and the importance of connecting regularly with at least one trusted friend during this time.

I could not imagine thrusting a book about kicking ass or crushing goals into this hurting woman's hands.

As the nurse drew blood to fill a few small vials, I leaned against the exam table and waited. Blood gurgled through the little plastic tubing, and Maureen looked up at me, her face brightening. "You want to hear something strange?"

"Sure," I said, nodding.

"It just feels good knowing he's safe right now. He's safe in the hospital, you know? And last night after group therapy, we played Scrabble together. He beat me, of course. And he laughed and teased me. He was just the same person he's *always* been. And he seemed . . . happy."

She stopped then, and her eyes appeared to be far away, searching. "It was this beautiful moment with him. In a *hospital*. Isn't that a strange thing to say?"

I smiled. Life is so bittersweet.

The nurse left the room, and Maureen gathered her things, shoved her phone and old, rumpled Kleenexes back into her purse, and stood. I held my arms open to give her a hug. As she pulled away from our embrace, I pointed gently toward her pants and said, "Hey Maureen, take as long as you need. But it looks like you've got your joggers on inside out. You might want to change them around before you head back out there. You can come see me anytime you need to, but let's make a follow-up appointment for two weeks."

She looked down at her pants, at the white cotton pockets sticking out from her hips, then back at me, realizing she'd been walking around all morning with her pants on inside out. Her eyes sparkled and danced for a moment as we both burst into laughter.

Life is hard, isn't it? Especially in this middle place. One thing I know for certain is that women *are* weary. We long to "kick ass" in midlife and "crush all our goals." But then life happens. Our marriages fail, our children grow and change and we send them out into the pain of the real world where they must live very real lives, we lose jobs, we lose loved ones, our parents age and decline and require more help, our own bodies tire and our hormones begin playing tricks on us.

We simply . . . struggle. And though the Christian publishing industry seems to prefer "prescriptive" type books and I *am* a family practice doctor well-versed in writing prescriptions, I simply don't have a tidy prescription to offer for all the complexities women face in midlife.

One of the challenges of this book is how to wear my "expert" hat and offer my medical expertise while also being truthful about my own personal struggles. I want to tell you everything I know about women's bodies and medicine and healing, but I also want to be real about what is hard and broken and painful. After all, I counsel women on their health and general well-being, but at the same time, I sometimes eat from the huge bag of Ruffles in my pantry. Somehow, my medical knowledge doesn't prevent me from struggling with anxiety and unhealthy body image, adult acne and weight gain, or the heavier periods that can be typical of our mid-forties.

I am weary, too.

* * * *

Years ago, on my surgery rotation during residency, the head surgical nurse leaned over before the next scheduled surgery of the day and nodded toward the cardiothoracic surgeon. "He doesn't usually let the residents scrub in on these procedures, you know. He must like you."

I felt a mixture of pride and bewilderment. Ever the hard worker, I'd been striving for weeks to be dependable and knowledgeable on rounds—thorough, punctual, confident. But what in the world was I doing scrubbing in on a cardiac bypass grafting (CABG) procedure? It's not like I could lend any real help.

I watched it all with awe anyway.

The team began by harvesting a vein from the patient's leg to be used for a new blood vessel to the heart since the original cardiac arteries had become blocked with plaque over the years, inhibiting the supply of oxygen to the heart muscle and causing symptoms of a heart attack. Then, after they cut swiftly through the sternum with a little round bone saw, I watched as that head surgeon inserted a large metal retractor into the chest. It had a turn crank attached like those little wind-up toys that hop along on plastic legs or roll by themselves on the floor. "Want to take a few turns?" he asked. I heard the ribs crack a little wider with each twist of my wrist, slowly revealing the patient's lifeless heart underneath. During a CABG, the blood required by the body pumps through an elaborate cardiopulmonary bypass machine that mechanically exchanges the fresh oxygen needed to sustain all the body's tissues while the heart lies still and quiet in the chest.

To me, these miracles of science are simply concrete evidence of the Divine.

The surgeon paused then and looked up at me, his rich brown eyes squinching as he smiled beneath his blue surgical mask. "Have you ever held someone's heart in your hands?"

I shook my head no.

He grabbed my hands and wrapped my slippery gloves with gauze for some traction, then gently pulled the heart up and slightly out of the chest. "Here. Hold the heart *right here* and don't move. Keep your fingers flat, like this. If you hold too light, the heart will slip and rip the vessels, which will ruin the graft. If you hold too tight, your fingers will poke a hole right through the heart."

No pressure, right? On top of that, once he began the delicate process of stitching the freshly harvested vessels into place, I couldn't see a thing. I just stood there sweating for what felt like an eternity with a human being's heart in my hands. Literally holding on for dear life—not too light but not too tight. It was both exhausting and exhilarating. And, thankfully, the surgery was a success. The graft took. Our patient's blood began pumping once again through the heart that had been carefully laid back within the chest cavity. Then we wired his sternum closed with thick metal wire and stitched the remaining layers of muscle and skin gently over the top. I felt like I'd witnessed a modern-day miracle. And after work, I went home and told my husband with awe, "I got to hold someone's actual heart in my own two little hands today. Can you believe that?"

"That's amazing. Bet you won't ever get to do *that* again!" was his reply.

But he was wrong. Because that's exactly what I did in the clinic that day with Maureen. It's what I do with all my patients, really. Or with the readers who send messages after reading my first book or write to share pieces of their own story after relating to an online essay I've published. It's what I do for the friends I walk with through the neighborhood. Or for my best girlfriends over the phone. Turns out, I *often* hold another human being's heart in my hands. And that's exactly what I'm hoping to do with this book. I'm asking you to put your big, beautiful heart in my hands for a little while, and in return, I will offer you *all* of mine.

If you came as a patient into the clinic, I might get one or two fifteen- or thirty-minute appointments to talk with you every six months or so, which means it might take well over a year for me to get just an hour of your time and attention. And it isn't enough. It isn't enough time to look into your eyes and listen well and understand and really get to know you—who you are, what you're facing, where you come from. It isn't enough time to tell you all the things I long to tell you. It isn't enough time to even begin to find *true* healing. But here, now, and for the next 250+ pages, we have all the time we need. We can hold each other's hearts—not too light and not too tight—while we work toward healing in this messy middle part of our lives. Together.

* * * *

What you're reading here is *more* than a typical "Women's Health" book because women are *more* than menstruation and fertility and menopause. We are so much *more* than our reproductive organs and the outward appearance of our bodies. We are hearts and minds and flesh and bones and bowels and bellies and breasts and sex and love and fire and rage and joy and whole entire lives all folded and forged into one uniquely beautiful God-given form. Not *every* problem that arises for a woman in midlife can be chalked up to hormones or menopause. Instead, we must consider our age and other medical issues including medications or supplements if we take them, our diet and exercise and sleep patterns, our underlying genetics, our history of trauma, our experiences and current stressors, any socioeconomic stressors or discriminatory barriers, plus our ability to provide self-care and lean on appropriate support systems if they are available to us. Midlife is complicated, and our midlife bodies are certainly complex! What is considered healthy for one woman may be substantially different from what is considered healthy for another. So, during this phase of life we must make informed decisions and work together with our medical providers to develop treatment plans or lifestyle modifications *based on the whole picture unique to each one of us.*

What I'm sharing with you in the pages that follow are real heart stories about love and truth and life. Stories of pain and hurt and motherhood and marriage and faith and friendship entwined. Of struggle and strain and renewal and hope combined with our health and healing along the way. I'm confident you'll see a part of yourself here in one or more of these stories. And my hope is that not only will you learn something new about your body or caring for your health during this middle part of life's journey, but also you will take to heart the truth that you're not alone in a single moment of this good, hard, ordinary life.

What follows is everything I wish I could tell you about midlife.

Each chapter will begin with a true-life event from a patient I've treated in clinic or a friend I've listened to on a long walk around the path by my house or from the very *real* issues I've faced in my own life. And each chapter will conclude with pertinent medical information on a wide range of topics women routinely encounter in their later thirties, forties, fifties, and beyond along with tools to empower you to care for and heal the body you *actually* have (rather than the utterly impossible cultural ideal—ugh, more on that later).

We'll talk about the slippery subject of control, shame-based "health" practices vs. love-based healing, how to evaluate our readiness for change, and the importance of forming deep relationships with the team God sends to offer help and love and connection in our lives. I'll bring scientific insight to your burning medical questions about the thyroid and symptoms of adult attention deficit hyperactivity disorder (ADHD) and the unexpected rage of premenstrual dysphoric disorder (PMDD) and perimenopause and various mood disorders like generalized anxiety and depression. We'll discuss the preventive healthcare measures applicable to you in your current life stage as well as dietary supplements that can offer additional support. I will give scientific definitions as well as additional resources for further reading and learning. And I hope to provide a jumping-off point for further conversations with your personal medical provider about your own specific situation and the parameters of your particular body.

My great hope with this book is that together we can open our brave, battered, beautiful hearts to God's love and grace and mending and mercy, accepting that this one precious life we're living *is* hard, especially in this middle place. As women we often feel weary, and I certainly cannot promise that the best of life is yet to come. But there *are* steps we can take toward health and healing in these precious bodies we've been given while discovering (often surprisingly) along the way . . . there is beauty *here*, too.

1

PROMISES OF THE "BEAUTY AND WELLNESS" INDUSTRY

I am sitting at a folding table in the gathering hall at Holy Spirit Catholic Church. It is my first time participating in Sunday school. I must attend for six weeks to receive the sacrament of reconciliation followed by my first communion. And, as a third grader, I am already one year behind, a whole grade older than all the others.

The teacher is calling out names and chapters and numbers from the front of the room while all the second graders sitting around me are racing through their personalized children's Bibles with monogrammed leather covers to find the right page. In a matter of seconds, their little hands go shooting into the air as they holler with pride "I found it!" or "I win!"

I have no idea what anyone is doing. But I pretend. I pretend to know.

My stubby-nailed fingers flip quickly through the thin pages of the borrowed Bible I picked up from the front table when I entered the room, and I notice some familiar names at the top. Isaiah. Luke. John. *Yes, I think I've heard of those.* But the other kids are lightning fast, and I lose again and again and again. I don't understand the books or chapters or numbers the teacher is calling. I'm not aware of the difference between the Old and New Testament. *There's an order to this? A reason?* I don't understand. But I must attend classes for six weeks so I can receive the sacrament of first communion (which comes with the added bonus of a fancy certificate with scrolly lettering . . . that part I understand). I must flip pages. I must pretend to race against the others and then pretend to be disappointed when *Oops! So close! I almost had it but . . . I've failed again.*

Next the teacher smiles and asks if anyone can recite the Beatitudes, and I shove the nail of my index finger into my mouth and nervously rip the end away, drawing blood. There seems to be something here that everyone else understands. A point. And when we practice the prayer for reconciliation, I already know what I will say when it is my turn alone with the priest. "Bless me, Father, for I have sinned. This is my first confession. I don't understand my life. I'm not sure what I'm supposed to be doing here. And I have no idea how I'm supposed to fix any of it."

I would spend the next few decades of my life trying.

We *long* to fix our lives, don't we? It's a deep desire that takes root in our minds because from the beginning, we are endlessly force-fed two illusions by the world. The first is that we can construct a life without difficulty or pain, that life should be easy and happy and simple (maybe even a bit polished and shiny). And that there *is* some destination toward which we should all be heading. The second is that if we plan and work hard enough and arrange all the pieces just so and follow all the rules, then we can control the outcome. No matter what happens in life, there is something we can *do* about it. *Everything is fixable.*

The world holds out promises like a fistful of bright yellow dandelions from the side of the road. They are so cheerful and pretty that we believe them and all their happy beauty . . . at first.

But with time, the bright yellow blooms wilt and fade. We glance down from the wilted blooms in our hands to the dandelion patch they came from and notice its green tendrils spreading out and taking root down below. The lush green grass underfoot is beginning to thin, and suddenly we're struck with doubt. *Wait. Are these flowers or weeds?* We blow our wishes on the white fluff anyway and watch it go dancing through the breeze. We wonder if this is all there is. *Shouldn't there be . . . more?* And it seems like ages before fresh, bright yellow blooms spring up from the seeds like unlikely new hope.

Are the world's promises flowers or weeds? I'm still not really sure. But the wellness industry promises us there is an answer. A quick Google search of "wellness" or "simple living" or "how to have a healthy life" yields thousands upon thousands of book titles like:

- Designing Your Life: How to Build a Well-Lived, Joyful Life
- Build Your Life from the Inside Out
- The Life You've Always Wanted
- Essentialism: Regain Control of Health, Well-being, and Happiness
- Next Level: Your Guide to Kicking Ass, Feeling Great, and Crushing Goals through Menopause and Beyond

And it all sounds great to me. I'd love to regain control! Maybe even kick a little ass and crush some goals. *Can I really have the life I've always wanted? What do I do? What are the steps?*

We're told there is an algorithm to life, a best path, a *right way*, so from the beginning, we attempt to follow it. We buy into the world's promises and embrace these absolutes because our alternative is to face reality, and often, reality hurts. Instead, we clutch at the many lists of instructions thrown our way from parents and teachers and grown-ups and media and marketing and the world, and we begin chasing the arrows from box to box. We achieve. We pretend. We prove. And we attempt to build a *good* life.

First, the world tells us to strive. Do more, be more, have more! You're not doing it right unless you do it *all*. Achievement equals success and success equals happiness. So, get out there and go for it! You can be your best you! *This* is the meaning of life! And though it feels a lot like chasing an optical illusion, a mirage, or a rainbow (or, more likely, consumerism), we do our best to attain the perfect family, career, house, and stuff. We run half-marathons and restrict our diets. We weigh less, and we make more money. We buy things. We take beautiful family portraits and plaster them to the living room wall. And, more importantly, we post about it. *See? Look at me! I am winning at life today!*

But it isn't too far into living that we realize, rather unfortunately, we were born as imperfect humans on our very first day, and we cannot possibly win this losing game. The worldly ideal toward which we've been striving continually morphs and changes over time, making it impossible to ever cross the proverbial finish line. We cannot possibly meet the expectations of our parents and teachers and coaches or of social media and marketing and the world because that *thing* we've been continually chasing—worldly success and the cultural ideal of health, beauty, and wellness—will always be just the littlest bit out of reach.

On top of that, life happens.

We struggle with addiction or divorce, job loss or chronic illness, family feuds, infertility, infidelity, miscarriage, or death of a loved one. All those pieces we've been clutching so tightly in our fists and fumbling to arrange in just the right way begin to crumble to dust in our hands. And we are *so tired*. We have been building and acquiring and striving all this time, trying to follow the world's impossible algorithm, but suddenly we forget the point. *Wait . . . what is it all for?* We long for grace and rest and renewal, but the pain and bewilderment of life combined with the relentless empty promises of the "wellness" industry and the world aren't quite enough for us to stop. So instead of stepping out of the impossible game, we double down and try a new approach.

Surely the answer is out there. Somewhere.

Next, the world tells us to simplify. Pare down, declutter, live simply! You're not doing it right unless life feels free and easy. It really shouldn't be as hard as you're making it seem. Life should be simple, and the answers are right here. Remember? Everything is fixable! So, we attempt to solve it all over again. We buy a book on Whole 30 and download a meditation app to our phone. We move homes, switch jobs, downsize. We eat locally sourced foods, become vegan, take up yoga, live "tiny," whip up another smoothie and pop our earbuds into our ears, all while we breathe deep and practice mindfulness. We read articles about essentialism, we embrace minimalism, we buy self-help books with all those wonderful titles and amazing promises and serene photos on the cover. We feed the $4.4 trillion "beauty and wellness" industry[1] more of our hard-earned money as we continue counting and sorting and measuring and deserving, trying to make it all add up while quietly wondering, *Will I ever get the mix right? What is the point? And will ANY of this make me . . . well?* It's a culture that permeates everything and poisons everyone. I know because it poisons me, too.

❋ ❋ ❋ ❋

The primary victims of the "beauty and wellness" industry are women. Hoping to sell us more products and keep us constantly off-kilter and unfulfilled (and, oh by the way, make as much money as possible from our struggles), the marketing strategy for this ever-growing industry specifically targets our *pain points*—our motherhood and weight, our "sexiness" and relationships, our very normal and inevitable aging and changing appearance, our increasingly wrinkled and crepe-papery skin, and our sagging sense of self-worth. Using "science" and money and manipulation, the wellness industry promises to solve all our problems with some great new product or program that will make us happier and healthier and younger and thinner and just that much closer to living our "best life."

The wellness industry says, "We know you're struggling. You're tired and overwhelmed and stressed out . . . but don't *worry*, we have a product for that, a book for that, an injection for that, a diet for that, an exercise program for that, a supplement for that, a cleanse for that, a face cream for that, a smoothie recipe for that. You'll be prettier and younger and more energetic and thinner and probably waaaay more successful. Because remember? Today forty is the new thirty, fifty is the new forty, and *everything is fixable*. Now here, buy this. It's all natural! And your happiness is only one purchase away."

The wellness industry's empty promises coupled with the world's constant pressure to perform and improve—to be joyful in our motherhood, to be effortless in our sexiness, to be strong in our boss-babe careers, to be ever cognizant of our self-care, to be endlessly thin and young and organized and efficient and healthy and perfect, to seemingly do it ALL yet also manage to keep it simple—adds to the general weariness of life and can be absolutely lethal to our sense of true Self, to our *whole*ness. Turns out, we cannot be perfect. We cannot do it all. Life often *isn't* simple. And we will not ever achieve the "ideal" being sold to us through the "beauty and wellness" industry's marketing because it's a lie.

I wonder . . .

- Can we stop striving toward the costly "wellness" mirage that seems to move ever farther away the faster and harder we run toward it?
- Can we take ourselves off the hook of achieving the cultural ideal, and instead, live this very *real* life the best way we know how?

- Can we embrace this complex middle part of life as a time for change, deep growth, and continued learning?
- Can we set ourselves free to experience delight in our complicated, tumultuous lives—even right *in the middle* of the hard?
- Can we take ourselves out of the world's losing game and begin to fully love, care for, and gently heal the beautifully imperfect bodies we *actually* have? Can we find and embrace our true Self?

Focused primarily on power and money and wealth, the "beauty and wellness" industry seems to care very little about who we really are in our uniquely precious and beautiful lives. But here's something revolutionary: What if *we* did? Let's begin here and learn to cut through the noise.

Digging Deeper into Science

Before we go any farther into this book or discuss medical conditions specifically affecting women in the middle part of our lives, let's talk about science by looking at a few important definitions:

- **Normal** means conforming to a type, standard, or regular pattern; normal is considered usual or routine among the general population; it's a state of being without underlying pathology.
- **Common** means occurring or appearing frequently.
- **Ideal** refers to a standard of perfection, often taken as a model for imitation in the culture at large.[2]

These terms are often used interchangeably but really, they shouldn't be. Something can be a common condition (like being nearsighted and requiring glasses or contacts for correction) but not necessarily normal since there is an underlying pathology. Or something can be a normal phenomenon (like having stretch marks after childbirth or a roll around the middle during perimenopause) but not even close to the wellness industry's picture of ideal. Often, marketing will point to normal variances in the human form and lead us to believe we need to do something to "fix" them. As we move forward in this book, let's remember a thing can be normal or common and not necessarily need any intervention even if it does not fit the cultural ideal.

Let's also remember a thing can be normal or common and not necessarily apply to *you*. For example, the average woman is 5'4" and weighs 170 lbs., but those numbers may not be accurate for *you*.[3] It doesn't mean the science is wrong or those averages are wrong or there's anything wrong with you. We just need to remember that every human being is unique. Science is science and supported by time and research and data, but it turns out, science is often not exactly an *exact* science, especially when applied to an individual.

So, how do we know what to believe?

I'm still proposing we follow the science and rely on something called evidence-based medicine, which uses a systematic approach. These days, we hear a lot about "doing your own research," but unless someone has a laboratory set up in their basement with test subjects and controls and all the rest, they are more than likely "reading a lot about *other people's* research" and then drawing their own conclusions. In fact, this is what doctors do every day. We rely on layers and layers of credible research done by hundreds of thousands of scientists and researchers that has been collected and expanded upon over decades (centuries!) of time. Some call this "cookbook" medicine, but really, isn't that reassuring? If you're baking a cake, regardless of the flavor, doesn't it require a rising agent? Similarly, in medicine we tailor a treatment plan for the individual patient, but we devise that plan from a generally agreed upon standard of care based upon previous credible research.

Now the question becomes: whose research do we listen to? And how do we know if that research is *credible*? We hear many, many stories about what worked for our neighbor's boss's aunt, for example. Or even what so-and-so had to say about the terrible thing that happened to her grandmother. And, unfortunately, viral TikTok videos can be very enticing and entertaining. But . . . what does *science* have to say?

Let's define the difference between anecdotal evidence and empirical evidence and look at the importance of randomized double-blinded placebo-controlled trials to understand how medicine relies on evidence-based research to generate a gold standard of treatment for the disease processes of humans.[4]

- **Anecdotal evidence** is evidence in the form of stories people tell about what has happened to them that are passed along to others without the support of true scientific data. Associations may be made and may even have some merit, but until a clinical trial is performed it can only be taken at face value—"This is what worked for my neighbor's boss's aunt." It should be noted that sometimes these associations are how credible research and clinical trials begin. *Hmmm . . . maybe we should study that?*

Unfortunately, the spread of anecdotal evidence through mainstream media (who love to play on the general population's fear) and social media (who may have a vested interest in gaining more followers or selling a product) can contribute to something called the **illusory truth effect**,[5] which is the idea that the more times we hear something, the more accurate we believe it to be. Even if there is absolutely no science to back it.

- **Empirical evidence** is evidence based on both real-world observations and the data collected through scientific studies, which may include experimental studies, observational studies, clinical trials, surveys or interviews, and comparative analysis. Empirical evidence is used to create solid theories that can then be broadly applied to the general population.

- **Randomized double-blinded placebo-controlled trials** are experimental studies in which one group of subjects is randomly selected to receive the "real thing" (the active substance being tested) and the other half is randomly selected to receive a **placebo** (a substance designed to look like the real thing but that has no medical properties, often termed the "sugar pill"). It's termed "double-blinded" because neither the participants nor the researchers are aware of which treatment or intervention participants are receiving until the clinical trial is over, making results of such studies less likely to be biased. Results of such studies are said to be "evidence based."

- **Evidence-based medicine** is a systematic approach toward individual patient care often through set algorithms that doctors and other health care professionals follow based on the best available scientific evidence from empirical evidence tested through randomized double-blinded placebo-controlled trials and ongoing clinical research.

- **The Gold Standard** is the "best practice" in medicine widely accepted as being the best available test, intervention, procedure, or course of treatment for a given disease based on the results of multiple randomized double-blinded placebo-controlled trials. A gold standard is what would be used in a court of law during litigation proceedings after an undesirable outcome in medicine. This is what "the experts" have to say about best practices in medicine.

Are there caveats to following the science? Yes, of course! A medical study in and of itself is not comprehensive. Instead, it is meant to be used as a tool to help us understand and assess potential diagnostic and treatment options. It can't include *all* the information about certain conditions, treatments, medications, side effects, and risks that may apply to a specific patient. It cannot substitute for the medical advice, diagnosis, or treatment from a health care provider based on an examination and the assessment of a particular patient's specific and unique circumstances. When looking at the science, it is important to stop and ask yourself: *How does the science apply to me and the very particular parameters of my life, background, genetics, risk factors, and current situation?*

While I believe most medical researchers have everyone's best interest at heart, there are occasions when the wellness industry uses our pain points for exploitation and an attempt to make money (remember, the beauty and wellness industry is a $4.4 trillion industry). A "study" you find on the internet may use a lot of science-y terms and convincing statistics and sound pretty legit, but then actually turn out to be a steaming pile of, ummmm, bologna. So, how can we tell?

Here are questions you can use to help determine the validity and reliability of any "scientific" study:[6]

1. Why was the study done? What is the specific question it is attempting to answer?

2. Who conducted the study? Do they have the appropriate training and expertise?

3. Who funded the research? Was it sponsored by a third party? Or is there a vested interest in the results?

4. How was the data collected? Be sure to pay attention to the sample size and makeup of the population studied—a larger and more diverse sample size is necessary in order for a study to be applied universally to a larger audience and the general public.

5. Does the research *actually* measure what it claims? Did it measure the question? Be leery of any jumps (or gigantic leaps) from the results into associations. Do those associations even make sense?

6. Can the findings correctly be generalized to a larger population?

It's helpful if the study has been peer-reviewed, meaning it has been evaluated by physicians and scientists well versed in the particular topic. Ask yourself, *Do other experts in the field agree with the methods and findings? How do the study's conclusions fit with other studies in that area?* Be leery of any supplements with a doctor or scientist's face plastered to the front or any "study" with links to buy a line of products or "pay out of pocket" type treatments at the end. There is bound to be bias there.

Finally, I'll remind you that research is ongoing, and science is ever-changing. We as humans feel comforted by certainty, but in the medical field especially, we are constantly learning what works better now or what we were wrong about just a few years ago. What we believe to be true today could eventually change as more research and empirical evidence becomes available. So let's agree to make decisions based on the best available truth from reputable studies at this current moment in time.

In many ways, the wellness industry routinely lies to us. There *is* no "right way" for living a perfect life, and everything is *not* fixable. Green smoothies, "healthy" cleanses, "natural" supplements or not, our marriages will change, our children will grow, we will lose loved ones, our parents will age, and our own bodies will tire and age. We *will* struggle. And I regret to inform you we are all going out the same way.

But there *is* good news.

Just for today, we are here. We are alive, we are breathing, and we are imperfectly *human*. Our lives are both ordinary and magical. And when we stop endlessly chasing the world's definition of "beauty" and "wellness," we can be free to startle awake to the stunning everyday beauty of our good, hard, ordinary lives and the magnificence of the world all around.

This is how we *truly live*.

Focus on Healing

Listen, it might be your thyroid . . . but perhaps your symptoms are further complicated by the incredible mental load of motherhood. It could be adult ADHD . . . but your inattention is likely all muddled up with the gargantuan list of unattainable expectations placed on women in our society to do it *all*. It might be PMDD . . . but what if the unresolved marital issues you stuffed away years ago are also playing a role? It could be depression or anxiety or some other similar mood disorder . . . but perhaps it's time to come face to face with the childhood trauma you've been dragging along with you through life. And yes, it might be related to hormones and perimenopause . . . but I would venture to guess you're also drowning in the emotional exhaustion of simply being a woman in midlife—the endless lists, the grocery shopping, the barrage of emails, the constant attempts to balance your work life with your home life, the doctor appointments and dentist appointments and optometrist appointments, plus the fundraiser for soccer, weeknight dinners around everyone else's schedules, ACT exams and driver's ed courses, your aging parents, and the never-ending worry about whether or not your teenage son is texting (or drinking) while he's driving.

Perhaps you'd feel a little better if you followed a healthy(ish) diet and found time for regular exercise and made space in your day for self-care and took the appropriate supplements and prioritized your sleep. These are, of course, very reasonable suggestions. In fact, I recommend them! But as we move forward together through this book, I'd like to remind you to give yourself a hefty daily dose of grace for being *exactly where you are* in a life *just exactly like this*. We are living inside difficult and complicated bodies walking around in very difficult and complicated lives. Life is simply *hard*. And it doesn't mean you're doing it wrong; it means you're *living a life*.

Throughout this book I'll provide you with true stories AND science to reassure you that you're likely normal, you're definitely not alone, and there are many ways to live a healthier life into your forties, fifties, and beyond without endlessly chasing the $4.4 trillion "beauty and wellness" industry's picture of ideal. *This* is the path to real healing.

2

SO, *COULD* IT BE
YOUR THYROID???

After four years of undergraduate work for a bachelor of science degree in biology and four years of medical school for a doctorate, I completed three years of residency in family practice followed by one year of fellowship training specifically in women's health. Now, after nearly two decades practicing in general family practice, I can say I've treated thousands of women in this midlife stage going through infinite versions of the same thing—changing family dynamics, newly horrendous periods, low energy and poor concentration, the struggle to rebalance work and personal life due to shifting motherhood and midlife roles, financial concerns or marital problems, physical complaints due to chronic daily stress or grief or medical illness, and a dull inexplicable rage simmering just below the surface.

In the face of life's co-occurring stressors, many of us are asking for answers:

- Is it my thyroid? Or maybe a brain tumor?
- Do you think I might have adult ADHD because I can't seem to finish a single thought and I just walk around the house all day forgetting why I walked into the room?

- Why am I so tired all the time?
- Am I the only mother questioning every parenting decision I've ever made because the kids are suddenly so sullen and quiet?
- Is this just midlife hormones? Or could it be menopause?
- Oh, and do you think it's normal to cry so much? Do you think it's normal to have so much rage?

Dr. Albertson, is this *normal*? Often my patients' eyes are pleading, *The world promised me more. And I always thought life would be more beautiful than this. Can you fix it? Will you fix . . . me?*

I wait, then listen and reassure them, "Sure, I can check your thyroid. And I'll add a complete blood cell (CBC) count and an iron level to check for anemia. Are you taking calcium with vitamin D? Let's add a vitamin D level to your blood work. Plus, a blood sugar level to rule out prediabetes. How often do you exercise? And how's your diet? Tell me about your periods. And your sleep schedule. Then maybe let's discuss your mood in a little more detail."

When their blood work comes back normal, and it *isn't* a thyroid problem or iron-deficiency anemia or low vitamin D or some wacky hormone level, I might discuss a trial of a selective serotonin reuptake inhibitor (SSRI) for anxiety or depression, a regular exercise program that includes resistance training, a daily multivitamin, more water intake, plus a few sessions of therapy or perhaps some form of menopausal hormone therapy (MHT). And I can see the flicker of defeat in their eyes. They've heard this before, and I always wish I could do more. I'm offering a few Band-Aids when really, what we *all* so desperately need is restoration and peace—we need deep connection and full lives and true healing and unconditional love for the precious, beautiful lives and bodies we *actually* have.

When you come as a patient to my clinic and your eyes are defeated and pleading—*Can you fix it? Will you fix me?*—more than anything, I want to put my stethoscope down and take you gently by the hands and tell you:

I don't know if I can fix this, but I know more than you think I do. I know you've been stewing over this appointment for months. Putting it off. Avoiding the call because it's hard to schedule anything for yourself into the day—a day filled with dishes and laundry and kids' lunch boxes and errands and expectations and work emails and after-school homework and a hard phone call from your mother and all the baggage you're silently carrying from childhood and soccer practices and carting someone home from driver's ed and dinner and bath time and bedtime and that last kitchen clean-up of the day. Plus, you're nervous about what must be wrong with you because you're so tired all the time that it feels like you can't get anything accomplished.

I know it took a huge effort for you to get here. You had to rearrange your morning schedule and wake everyone a little early and drop the kids at school with pretty pathetic-looking lunches (Bento boxes? Umm . . . no. Not in your house). And after this appointment and a few errands, you're hoping to get home in time to grab something to eat and get some work done on the computer before school finishes. You work from home now while also attempting to shuttle kids back and forth from school and to practices because the afterschool program costs are atrocious. Plus, you feel all the pressure to make sure the kids are "well-rounded." You look forward to this small sliver of quiet time every single day, and you are annoyed I am running twenty minutes behind. Now you'll never get it all done before it's time to pick up the kids!

I know you fixed yourself up before you came. In hopes of looking a bit more "put together," you showered and fixed your hair and put on makeup. You even wore a cardigan because years ago Glennon Doyle said "good" moms who are "put together" probably wear cardigans (she was being sarcastic and funny, except I know you still kind of believe this theory).[1] And I know you're not sure what to say. When I walked into the room just now, a tiny voice in the back of your mind whispered, *Why did I even come here? She doesn't understand. She has no idea what I'm going through.*

41

And she's probably not going to be able to help me, anyway. I should just get up and leave!

But I also know you don't feel well.

You just don't feel right. And you are tired ALL. THE. TIME. You're not hungry or you're too hungry and no matter what you do, you seem to be gaining weight (this is the second new pair of jeans you've upsized this year!). You can't sleep at night because your mind is racing, and during the day you repeatedly fall asleep at your desk or on the couch after work even though you have a ton of laundry to fold.

Your periods have changed. In your twenties you barely noticed having a period, but now, month after month your periods are a nightmare. The time between your cycles is shorter and your bleeding is longer and heavier, and you recently heard some woman on the soccer sidelines talking about menopause. You think to yourself, *Is this menopause? I'm forty-four! It's way too early for that, right?* Plus, you're so incredibly angry in the days leading up to your period that you scare yourself sometimes, and it haunts you. You never envisioned carrying this much rage. Then when your period starts, you can barely go out of the house because you soak through a tampon in less than two hours. During your period you walk around with the same terror you had in middle school, worried about blood on the back of your pants. And, also, you're wondering, *What is with this adult acne? Isn't acne for pubescent boys with raging testosterone and cracking voices?*

I know you're worried something is terribly wrong with you. Or you're worried nothing is wrong with you and you must just be crazy (then you feel guilty for using the word "crazy" because we're not supposed to say that these days). And I know you hope I can help. You're doubtful I can, but mostly, you hope it's your thyroid. You think, *It's got to be my thyroid, right? That would explain the weight gain and fatigue.* Plus, you hope I can give you medication to make you feel like a normal person—a person with some energy, a "happy" person. I know you feel guilty because some days you aren't happy, and you worry this means you are a terrible mom or a terrible spouse or just generally a terrible human, and you think, *But I have NOTHING to be unhappy about!*

You don't like it when I ask questions about depression or anxiety or mention anything about therapy (even though you quietly wonder about it yourself). You shush yourself constantly and think, *But I have NOTHING to be depressed about! Other people have it so much worse!*

I know you know you could be eating better and exercising and getting at least seven hours of sleep. I can see the defeat in your eyes when I ask about it because you tell yourself every day that you'll be better at all these things, that today is the day. *Today is the day I'm going to start eating well! Today is the day I'm going to start practicing self-care!* But then life gets in the way. Your youngest is sick and the older kids have an event at school and there are several sports practices or music lessons in one night, so you spend your evening in the car. Then your mom calls to tell you about her doctor's appointment and how she may need to have surgery next week and by the time you get off the phone taking down all the details so you can rearrange your schedule to help her out, you don't have time to get to the gym let alone cook a healthy meal. So, you end up with a drive-thru dinner for the whole family. Again.

And I know you beat yourself up about it.

You beat yourself up on a regular basis, in fact. You're convinced you are a horrible mom because you lost your temper with the kids again even though you are rereading your tattered copy of *Scream-free Parenting*. Or you believe you are an awful spouse because your husband repeatedly comes home to a tired wife and fighting children and a messy house and grilled cheese for dinner. Plus, you're so exhausted every night that having sex sometimes feels like another chore on the never-ending to-do list. You wonder, *Has it been three weeks since our last time? Or four? And should I care a little more about that? Are other couples having sex . . . more?*

If you stay home, you worry you should be working. Or working more. Or maybe if you are working full time, you worry you should be staying home. Or working part time so you can be around in the afternoon for the kids after school. Or at least making more money. Or perhaps for the first time all the kids are in school during the day, and you lose sleep wondering what you're supposed to do now. You are terribly worried that you might not be living your life's purpose. You think, *What is my life's purpose? Have I missed it? Maybe if I just had more energy . . .*

I get it. I feel that, too.

I know more than you think I do when you come with desperate tears in your eyes to tell me you don't feel well. And I want you to know some things, too. I want you to know I see you. I'm listening. I know you are struggling, and I want to help. I want so badly to fix it. More than anything in the world I want to help you feel better. It might be your thyroid, but it might be a whole slew of other possible disorders since symptoms like fatigue and decreased energy and dry skin and weight changes and poor concentration and diminished mood and insomnia and bowel changes and headaches could mean a vitamin deficiency or an autoimmune disease (like lupus or fibromyalgia or celiac disease or multiple sclerosis or a thyroid disorder) or some other endocrine tumor or sleep apnea or perimenopause or underlying substance abuse or depression or anxiety or simply the symptoms of being an overstressed, overtired woman carrying all the weight of the world's expectations right in the middle of midlife.[2]

I want to tell you I understand. And it may take some time to tease it all out. The International Classification of Diseases (IDC) has something like seventeen thousand unique codes for more than ten thousand known diseases. So, any one symptom may have dozens (or hundreds) of possible causes. I sure wish I had a little scanner to pass over each patient's wrist to see the precise diagnosis pop up on my computer screen. But as it is, I must begin with a series of questions, a physical exam, and an initial panel of blood work that I might need to expand upon later depending on the results. And honestly? I hope it's a thyroid problem, too. I hope I check a thyroid-stimulating hormone (TSH) level and find it through the roof and start some Levothyroxine; then when you follow up in four to six weeks, you tell me you feel like a new woman because you responded well to the starting dose of medication. I always hope to find an easy, tangible abnormality that I can likely do something about so you can feel better. I wish I had the answers for you. I wish I could fix it.

I've come to realize my passion in life, whether in the clinic with a patient or writing for my online community or talking to a girlfriend on the phone or walking around the path near my house with a neighbor, is seeing, listening to, and really hearing women. Really helping women heal. More than anything, I want healing for you.

I want healing, too.

So, let's start now. Let's start here. And, since many of us wonder if our symptoms of bone-aching tiredness and seemingly perpetual weight gain could be related to a thyroid problem, let's start with the thyroid. What do you need to know about the thyroid gland and thyroid disease?

Digging Deeper into the Thyroid

The thyroid is a butterfly-shaped gland in the front part of your neck that produces two hormones—**triiodothyronine** (**T3**) and **thyroxine** (**T4**)—and it works like a little motorized control valve for your body's metabolism, revving up or revving down or occasionally burning out completely.

The function of the thyroid gland is controlled by interactions between the hypothalamus and pituitary gland. The **hypothalamus** is an area in the brain that controls both the **autonomic nervous system** (in charge of temperature, thirst, hunger, sleep, emotional activity, and body homeostasis) and the pituitary gland. The **pituitary gland** is a small gland in the brain with a role in growth and development as well as the function of multiple endocrine glands including the thyroid through a hormone called **thyroid-stimulating hormone** (**TSH**). This intricate network between the hypothalamus, pituitary gland, and thyroid gland functions on a feedback loop to maintain a relatively constant and necessary level of circulating thyroid hormone for your body's weight, general energy level, and other functions.

Problems with your thyroid gland's function can arise within the little motor of the thyroid gland itself or from problems within its control circuits in your pituitary gland or the hypothalamus. When the thyroid gland revs up and kicks into overdrive, it is referred to as **hyperthyroidism**. When the gland slows down and sputters to a near stop, it is called **hypothyroidism**.

Up to 12% of the US population will develop a thyroid disorder in their lifetime, and stunningly, more than half of women with a thyroid disorder are left undiagnosed. Most thyroid disease is a result of **primary hypothyroidism** from Hashimoto's disease (also called autoimmune thyroiditis in which the body's immune mechanisms begin to attack its own tissue) and is more common in women, increasing in incidence with age.

Because the thyroid gland regulates the body's overall metabolism through its little rev-up-or-rev-down motor, a change in thyroid gland function causes symptoms related to changes in the body's metabolism and energy. Symptoms of thyroid dysfunction are notoriously nonspecific and can mimic the symptoms of other common conditions or the normal changes associated with aging. (Which is why we are constantly wondering if it could be our thyroid—*am I stressed, overtired, simply aging, or is this a thyroid problem???* It can be really hard to tell!)

Symptoms of hypothyroidism may include

- fatigue or decreased energy level
- slow thinking or "brain fog"

- weight gain
- constipation
- intolerance to cold temperatures or feeling cold all the time
- extreme tiredness or shortness of breath with exercise
- dry skin, thinning hair, and brittle fingernails

The diagnosis of thyroid disease is made by checking your blood levels of TSH, T4, and T3.

TSH numbers can be confusing because a *high* TSH value actually means an underfunctioning thyroid gland (imagine the pituitary gland in the brain sending out more TSH signal, telling the thyroid gland to get to work) while a *low* TSH value corresponds to an overactive thyroid. They are inversely proportional. A normal TSH level is 4 to 5 mU/L in most laboratories (these numbers can vary from lab to lab so each lab will provide its own reference range of normal), though some people who have clear symptoms of hypothyroidism with a seemingly normal TSH will still benefit from treatment. As part of a thyroid evaluation, your provider might recommend further blood work, which may include thyroid autoantibodies to evaluate for an autoimmune cause.[3]

Other types of thyroid conditions may need further work-up with imaging using an ultrasound or an iodide uptake scan. And if the pituitary gland is thought to be the cause of a low functioning thyroid (a term called **"secondary" hypothyroidism**), further laboratory work to test the levels of other hormones made by the pituitary gland or brain imaging may be necessary.[4]

Treatment for hypothyroidism

Unfortunately, there is no "fix" for an underactive thyroid. Instead, we treat primary hypothyroidism with lifelong thyroid hormone replacement therapy using daily oral medication. Typically, a medication called Levothyroxine, which is a synthetic form of T4, is used for thyroid replacement. Some clinicians prescribe a form of T3 in addition to T4; however, studies have not shown a clear benefit to this combination.[5] Once an appropriate level of TSH is achieved, occasional adjustments to dosages are based on regular intervals of laboratory monitoring at least every six months.

Yes, there are "natural" forms of thyroid replacement on the market. However, constant levels of thyroid hormones on these "natural" forms have been proven difficult to maintain, and those formulations are not routinely recommended. Furthermore, for several reasons I suggest you steer clear of "natural" products claiming to provide "thyroid support." We'll talk more about "natural" supplements in chapter 11.

Thyroid replacement medication should be taken once a day in the morning on an empty stomach since food or other medications can affect the absorption of T4. Other health conditions and medications may affect the dosage of thyroid medication needed to maintain a normal TSH and T4. It is important to ask your provider whenever you begin a new medication or are diagnosed with a new condition (including pregnancy) to see if your thyroid regimen needs to be adjusted.

There are many other forms of thyroid disease, including development of a thyroid goiter, thyroid cancers, hyperthyroidism, thyroid nodules, other types of thyroiditis or autoimmune disease of the thyroid, and more. Entire books have been written on the thyroid! Your healthcare provider is the best source of information for questions and concerns related to your thyroid.

Focus on Healing

As a physician, I understand you come to me looking for answers, and in many ways, I suppose I'm the expert. But really, I want you to know that we are on the same team. I long to appear "put together," but underneath the cardigan I threw on this morning, I'm struggling through my own life just like you. On any given day, it's likely I changed my pants five minutes after I got dressed because someone spilled an entire bowl of cereal on my lap at breakfast (leaving a soggy mess of milk in the laundry that I can look forward to dealing with later). Plus, after I finally went to bed last night (because, you know, teenagers), I woke up three times overnight. First to settle a sick kid back to bed, then to let our pestering cat out the back door, then to "cover me up real good." And that has been a fairly normal nightly routine for the last nineteen years running.

I am *so tired*, too.

Perhaps like me, you struggle a lot with the strange dichotomy of working and mothering. I know I often wonder, *Should I be working outside the home regularly? Or staying at home permanently? I went to school forever and we have so many student loans left to pay, but I love writing. And mothering. And helping others. There are so many things I want to DO with my short time here on earth. But what is my life's purpose? Have I missed it? Is this right? God, what is it I'm supposed to be doing here? What is the point?*

For years I had to baby-step my way into the office on workdays, telling myself, *Just go. The kids are fine! They have fun while you're away!* Then once I got there, I realized I'd rather skip the exam and take a long lunch with you, my patient, so we could *really* talk. Now I have the incredible privilege of writing to you instead.

So, here's one last thing I would tell you if you were a patient sitting across from me today:

Listen. If you have kids, I know you are a good mom. And if you're in a relationship, I'm confident you are a great spouse or partner. Plus, you're an amazing friend and a simply wonderful human. The whole idea of "life's purpose" we worry about? Well, we are both living it right now. Our "calling" is this messy, beautiful, ordinary life we're living today, this very moment. Sometimes it's simply hard to see the big picture from where we are today.

When your blood work returns, we might find something "wrong," or we might not. It might be your thyroid. Or your hormones and other labs might check out just fine. We might need to talk about healthy lifestyle changes or "normal" changes of midlife associated with the later reproductive years or perimenopause. And we might decide to try an antidepressant, hormone therapy, or other medication for symptomatic relief. It might take a few tries to find the right one followed by a few months to know if it's helping. I might suggest you see a therapist. Or I might refer you to a specialist because I just don't have the answer to what's going on.

I want you to know I do not think you are "crazy." You and me? We are not crazy. Life is simply hard! I know because I'm right here in the middle of it, too. There are so many transitions to navigate, so many unreasonable expectations whispering in our ears, so many new problems to walk through, so many hidden traumas we silently carry, and so much life going on all at once with a body that doesn't cooperate like it once did. And I wish I could fix it. I wish I had an easy answer or a prescription for the solution to all of it.

But unfortunately, this is the human condition. And being human is hard. There simply are no quick or easy solutions. But I want you to keep coming back, keep showing up, keep moving a few gentle steps forward toward love, better health, and healing. I believe we CAN find healing for our midlife bodies. We CAN discover purpose in our ever-changing roles as we enter new stages of life, marriage, motherhood, caregiving, relationships, and career. We CAN turn toward the hard, endless work of loving the only lives and bodies we've been given. And we CAN find beauty here, too.

We can do it together.

3

LET'S TALK ABOUT STRESS

I am learning for perhaps the thousandth (millionth?) time about life and faith and surviving this world's inevitable stressors, this time from two gorgeous women in my neighborhood. I meet them for walks on Monday mornings on the path by my house, where we take turns telling one another the truth of our lives.

We talk about the school's individualized education plans (IEPs) for our kids and what we found in our teenage son's room and the worries we carry about our husbands and the difficulties of raising a blended family and that terrible thing our mother said that made us want to cry like a child. Oftentimes we talk about Scripture and Jesus's undeniable presence in our lives. And sometimes my friend Angie shares about the neighbors she invites to her house for dinner or the seemingly endless number of people she teaches English to a few evenings a month—immigrant and non-English-speaking members of our neighborhood hoping to become more proficient in English and financial literacy and, basically, how to make a life in a foreign land. This beautiful, unassuming woman is one of the most genuine people I know.

Through tears, Angie recounts the hardships her students continue to endure, and the three of us walk along and talk and listen and sigh and wonder why life is so unfair. Why are some people asked to carry so much more than others? Why do some people lurch along through life facing one disaster after another? One heartbreak after another? One unfairness after another? Why do some people live a whole life with pain and loneliness and abuse and oppression and bitter financial constraints and, oh by the way, leukemia? And . . . what do those of us who have been seemingly #blessed do about it? How do we help?

Angie's lifework appears to be blessing other people, noticing the light from inside them that shines through the cracks and illuminates the darkness, then placing them high on a stand so the rest of us might bask in their rays. Except she doesn't know it. She would tell you she's "just" a stay-at-home mom. She would tell you she struggles to stay on task and get things done because of her scatterbrained ADHD mind. Instead of promoting or bragging about her good deeds and accomplishments or calling any attention to herself, she tends to prop up the amazing details of *everyone else's* lives and give all the glory to God while shoving her own beautiful attributes aside. She is generous and humble and faithful and kindhearted. And, right now, her father is battling an aggressive cancer.

He was diagnosed with malignant melanoma with metastasis to the lungs the week after her fiftieth birthday, which is spectacularly unfair because only a few years ago Angie lost her beloved mom to cholangiocarcinoma. The acute stress and trauma of possibly losing both parents to cancer within such a short time is layered upon the chronic stress of fulfilling a caregiver role—collecting details at doctor's appointments and driving to scheduled treatment infusions and helping her dad wherever she can—while still sifting through the aftermath of her mother's death. Plus, this new and unexpected caregiver role for her father has been thrown into the chaotic mix of raising four teenagers and taking care of a family and managing a household and helping her struggling neighbors and teaching evening English classes at church and *all* the rest. Angie is squished firmly within what's termed "the sandwich generation" in which women must care for both children and parents at once, and it's all layered with stress upon stress upon stress.[1]

It turns out, most people are struggling more than they will ever let on. I can't tell you how often someone goes to the doctor for a relatively minor complaint and suddenly, spontaneously breaks into tears as their current life tragedy spills forth. "I don't know why I'm telling you all this!" they say. Grown, seemingly successful men. Teenagers with a "whatever" attitude. The lonely grandmother estranged from her children. The polished and successful working woman. The put-together-appearing mom. The disheveled mom. (Most moms, actually.) So many people are struggling through something devastating. Plus, nearly everyone I know is still picking up the pieces in the aftermath of these last few tumultuous years.

One of the unexpected gifts of practicing medicine is that I've had a front-row seat to life. To people. To their struggles and challenges and hardships. I've seen people without all their protective outer layers, and what I've learned from this up-close-and-personal peek into other people's experiences and emotions and life stress and pain is that when you pick and peel away our sticky labels, we are all so much the *same* inside. Without the world's expectations and all our predetermined and oppressive labels like mother, father, grandmother, husband, wife, boss, sister, daughter, or friend, we simply become *human* instead.

Practicing medicine reminds me of our humanness. Our fallibility. Our frailty. Our finitude. And when I recognize and understand another person's humanness, I can sometimes begin to forgive my *own* humanness and remember to embrace my very own humanity—the ability to display compassion, kindness, understanding, generosity, tenderness, charity, and love. Because we are *all* so human, aren't we? When the exam room door closes solidly behind me, patients feel permission to put their worries in my hands for just a little while: "My sinuses are killing me and I just can't get over this cold, plus . . . um . . . I hate my job and I'm pretty sure my husband is having an affair!"

For that 10:15 a.m. time slot, patients feel safe to let go. Breathe. Cry. For fifteen- to thirty-minute increments, they can be loved and held. They can be fully, completely, imperfectly human, and the best I can do is simply sit and be human beside them. Often I can't help with their problems other than giving a prescription for amoxicillin and suggesting they squirt a bottle of nasal saline rinse up their noses. And often it's not a medical issue holding them down and pinning them to the ground, but rather, a series of disastrous life stressors gripping their hearts and sucking the breath from their chest (the sinus infection that brought them in was simply the final straw). I do my best to listen anyway. I wait. I provide space. I click a prescription through to the pharmacy. And I hold their unbearable pain firmly and tenderly in my hands for a while—not too light and not too tight—attempting to offer a few minutes of relief.

It's an understatement to say life is stressful, right? Though the details may differ significantly, whatever struggle you're going through is universal rather than exceptional. So, what can we do?

- What can we do in the face of cholangiocarcinoma and malignant melanoma that threatens to steal away our parents' lives all too soon?

- How do we survive the spontaneous combustion of a twenty-plus-year marriage to infidelity?

- Is there any way to relieve the unbearable pain of a broken relationship with our lifelong best friend over differences in religion or politics?

- How do we handle our constant daily interactions with a rude boss or coworker who always leaves us seething?

- And what about the vape pen that spilled out of our teenager's bookbag? Or the empty box of condoms we found in the drawer of his bedside table? Or the word *porn* popping up in the Google search history on the kids' iPad?

Add to that a pile of unpaid bills and the fact that our daughter is failing school and the hard truth that our younger son is desperate for orthodontia we probably can't afford. Not to mention that our email inbox is overflowing and it's time to register all the kids for school next year and Friday is someone's (which one again?) turn to be the star student of the week, which means we need to print pictures for an "All About Me" poster. Plus, we are out of milk. Again.

Life is a gigantic cesspool of stress, both the acute and chronic varieties. Sometimes acute stress looks like a sudden illness, an unforeseen accident, a recent change such as a job loss or a move across the country, or one teeny tiny, absolutely life-changing truth-bomb from a teenager. The explosion of whatever it is blows us out of the water. We just didn't see it coming. And in an instant, we feel the heat of panic and overwhelm rise in our chests.

Chronic stress, however, is the kind that simmers below the surface day after day—perhaps a chronic illness, daily marital disputes, financial difficulties, a challenging boss at work, or difficult relationships with extended family members—and much like the simmering and boiling black goo of a tar pit, that more insidious, chronic stress sucks our feet into place. We're stuck. And sinking. The result of chronic daily stress inside our bodies becomes a constant pressing against our organs and our souls that slowly leeches away our vitality and health until we can't fully breathe inside that pit.

So, what exactly happens inside our bodies when stress—both acute and chronic—weasels its way inside and begins wreaking havoc? And is there anything we can *do* about it?

Digging Deeper into the Stress Response

When an acute threat to safety occurs, the **amygdala**, which is the area of the brain responsible for the body's survival instincts and emotional processing, kicks on and sends a distress signal to the hypothalamus. The hypothalamus then alerts the body's **autonomic (think *automatic*) nervous system (ANS)**, which is in charge of our body's unconscious/involuntary processes like breathing, blood pressure, digestion, hormone release, the signal that we need to go to the bathroom, sexual arousal, and more. The ANS is further comprised of two parts:

1. The **sympathetic nervous system** presses on the gas to invoke our "fight or flight" response.
2. The **parasympathetic nervous system** acts as the brake to restore our "rest and digest" return to calm.

In response to distress signals sent from the amygdala, the sympathetic nervous system steps on the gas and stimulates the **adrenal glands** (a pair of glands situated atop the kidneys) to release catecholamines—**adrenaline** and **noradrenaline**—from the adrenal medulla along with **cortisol** from the adrenal cortex. And as a result, the body's heart rate increases, the blood pressure rises, and the breathing rate becomes more rapid. The pupils dilate. And the body's response to pain decreases. Blood glucose increases in the bloodstream through metabolic changes that cause the breakdown of stored carbohydrates in the muscle and liver, termed **glycogenolysis**, as well as the production of new glucose using amino acids in the liver, called **gluconeogenesis**. Certain vessels dilate, quickly shunting blood now rich with glucose and oxygen to the muscles to prepare for **fight or flight**.

At the very same time, similar distress signals from the amygdala also instruct the parasympathetic nervous system (remember, that's the brake) to become quiet. Energy and resources are diverted *away* from the areas of the body that don't contribute to immediate survival. The body's digestion slows, the immune/inflammatory response decreases, reproductive efforts take a back burner, and wound healing is delayed.[2]

Physical symptoms during an acute stress response may include

- Racing heart and palpitations (beats out of synch with the normal beating of the heart)
- Sweating or chills
- Nausea (often followed by diarrhea)
- Tunnel vision or muffled hearing
- Tremors and muscle twitching

The physiologic cascade of changes in the body initiated by the sympathetic nervous system in response to danger allows us to either turn and fight off the threat or run away as fast as we can to safety. However, a third response termed **freeze** may also occur. In this scenario, the brain quickly assesses that we are both too weak to fight and too slow to flee so the best option is to essentially "play dead." During a freeze response, the parasympathetic nervous system overrides the gas pedal of the sympathetic nervous system and throws on the emergency brake, leaving us to become immobilized and numb in the face of life-threatening danger.[3] Later we may wonder, *Why did I just stand there? Why didn't I kick and scream? Why didn't I fight back or run away?* But the truth is, our brain was doing the best it could to keep us safe in response to overwhelming events that seemed completely unsurvivable. Freeze is a dissociation tactic for survival that may leave a foggy memory of pain or trauma.

Pete Walker introduced a fourth response in his book *Complex PTSD: From Surviving to Thriving* called the **fawn response**. "A fawn response is triggered when a person responds to a threat by trying to be pleasing or helpful in order to appease and forestall an attacker," which is often the response chosen in the face of chronic trauma or abuse.[4]

Once a threat has passed and the body has effectively fought off the danger or run away to safety, the amygdala responds once again. The signals that revved up the sympathetic nervous system cease, and the parasympathetic nervous system begins to pump the brakes to slowly bring our heart rate, blood pressure, breathing rate, blood glucose, digestion, immune function, reproduction, and wound healing back to a level of **homeostasis**, or the stable balance that occurs between the body systems at times of safety and rest. Our body can once again return to a feeling of calm.

Following a freeze or fawn response, it can be common to experience feelings of panic, shame, or rage accompanied by a complex range of emotions like uncontrollable crying or seemingly inappropriate laughing. Some may experience physical symptoms like jitteriness, nausea, vomiting, or diarrhea as the parasympathetic nervous system releases the emergency brake and the body returns to homeostasis.

Generally, life stressors happen in cycles and our bodies respond accordingly—stress, response, calm, stress, response, calm. Unfortunately, we can't simply remain in a state of perpetual safety and calm. That's not how life works! And contrary to what we might think or feel at the time as our hearts pound and we try not to puke, our stress response system is actually *good* for us. Our bodies have a built-in automatic response to help us move through stressful states appropriately, keeping us safe and well despite the inevitable threats that come from living a very real human life.

It is important to note that stress and our response to life's inevitable stressors is very different than *trauma*. Trauma occurs when, despite the body's indwelling stress response designed to keep us safe, we feel completely overwhelmed and powerless in a stressful situation. When we feel alone, shamed, or unable to fully process the pain of an overwhelmingly stressful or terrifying situation, our resulting trauma can even lead to **complex post-traumatic stress disorder** (**PTSD**) characterized by flashbacks, nightmares, and often severe anxiety as well as other health problems.[5]

The **Adverse Childhood Experiences** (**ACE**) study done in the late 1990s evaluated the link between negative stressful and traumatic events in childhood and the resulting negative health outcomes in adulthood. The ACE study found that experiencing abuse, neglect, and extreme household challenges during childhood—domestic violence, parental abandonment, physical or sexual abuse, neglect or having a parent with mental illness, having an incarcerated family member, or substance abuse in the household—not only causes risk for diminished quality of life due to poor mental health, substance abuse, and personal risky behaviors, but also contributes to *all-cause* illness through alterations in gene expression and changes in brain development. The higher your ACE score from childhood, the higher your risk for later health problems including diabetes, heart disease, and auto-immune disease as an adult.[6] We'll talk more about the effects of trauma and how we can begin to heal in chapter 13.

Acute vs. chronic stress

Chronic stress works differently than acute stress because it keeps us locked in a prolonged heightened state of fight or flight. Over time, a chronically stimulated stress response can lead to feelings of irritability, frustration, and increasing desperation as the body inevitably fatigues. The resulting elevation in cortisol levels over a prolonged period of time can lead to depression by inhibiting our ability to experience pleasure.

The innate fight, flight, or freeze responses programmed into our bodies to keep us safe aren't necessarily appropriate to help process our repeated everyday stressors such as difficulties at work with a short-tempered boss, problems in a strained marriage, financial concerns, our surly teenager's behavior, the dirty looks of a grumpy neighbor, or one of a million other chronic stressors life throws our way. And instead of being able to complete the cycle through one of the body's innate responses—like punching our neighbor in the nose or hightailing it away from our angry boss—daily stress becomes pent up inside us without resolution, and we feel stuck.

This chronic stress and resulting fatigue in our bodies can result in poor concentration, an inability to complete tasks, frequent infections from decreased immune function, chronic high blood pressure and thus an increased risk for heart disease or stroke, chronic pain, increased risk for other chronic illnesses, and mood disorders such as generalized anxiety or depression.[7] To avoid the side effects of chronic stress being held in the body, we must learn to actively process *through* it.

Focus on Healing

Twins Emily Nagoski, PhD, and Amelia Nagoski, DMA, wrote an essential book about combatting chronic stress in our daily lives titled *Burnout: The Secret to Unlocking the Stress Cycle*. In it, they discuss the importance of "completing the cycle" after we experience a stressful event or after finishing yet another stressful day in a string of stressful days. They point out that our daily lives typically don't require us to fight off a lion or flee an offender, but instead, every day we confront moment after moment of plain old ordinary stress. At the end of the day, without completing the cycle of fight, flight, or freeze in our bodies, the physiologic cascade of events triggered by the amygdala and the sympathetic nervous system remains active and working. And as a result, we can feel the irritability and frustration build as our bodies fatigue under this heightened and stressed state. The Nagoski sisters propose we must consciously act to complete the cycle *ourselves* to return once again to a state of calm and rest. How? In their book, they provide helpful tools which I'll summarize here:[8]

Ways to complete the stress cycle

1. **Physical Activity**—Run or dance or swim or take a yoga class or follow the kids on a bike ride or do anything that gets your body moving and your lungs breathing deeply for somewhere around an hour a day. The Nagoskis claim

that "physical activity is the single most efficient strategy for completing the stress response cycle."[9]

2. **Deep Breathing**—Consider "box breathing" in which you complete several cycles of breathing in for a count of four, holding for a count of four, then exhaling for a count of four, and holding for a count of four. This breathing technique is especially helpful for relieving stress if you are also seated in a quiet space or lying flat on the floor and breathing from your belly with your eyes closed.

3. **Positive Social Interaction or Affection**—Meet up with a friend for dinner after work or schedule an evening walk with a neighbor or simply call your sister to rehash a few things during your drive home or after you tuck the kids into bed. A positive interaction with a loving person will remind you that the world is generally a friendly and safe space to be and, though life can be terribly hard, you are not alone here.

4. **Emotional Expression**—Process your emotions by allowing yourself to fully express them. Instead of quelling your natural response, let yourself experience a deep belly laugh or (equally as helpful) a big guffawing cry that leaves you hiccupping like a toddler.

5. **Creative Expression**—Write or paint or sing or make jewelry or work in the garden or bake or refinish a piece of furniture or spend any time at all creating something beautiful simply for the sake of creating something beautiful for the world.

You will know you've completed the daily stress cycle when you feel a shift in both your mood and body toward a feeling of calm, relaxation, and peace. You will stop thinking obsessively and replaying the events of the day. You will stop fidgeting with your hands and feeling like you'd rather go jump off a cliff than clean up after dinner. And you will begin breathing more deeply as the muscles in your neck, jaw, and shoulders relax. You will shift peacefully into a state of homeostasis.

The world is a stressful place, especially during these middle years. But we don't have to carry all the stress of our daily lives *inside us*. We can take positive steps to move through it and process our emotions, enlisting the help of a trained therapist if necessary, to complete the daily stress cycle.

My walks on Monday mornings with my beautiful neighbors along the path behind my house are just one way I work to complete the cycle of chronic stress in my life. Together with two dear friends, I get to talk about life and discuss Scripture and notice the evidence of Jesus in the everyday, ordinary moments, and in so doing, we complete the stress cycle *together*. We get a little exercise and actively listen and commiserate and share affection and express our emotions. And at the end of every walk, I know the three of us feel a little more calm, relaxed, and at peace.

You can do this, too. Simply choose a tactic from the above list every day to consciously complete the stress cycle and return once again to a state of calm and rest and bodily homeostasis. Then, exhale. Breeeeaaaaathe. You deserve peace.

4

HOW TO MOVE FORWARD WHEN LIFE GOES COMPLETELY OFF THE RAILS

Three industrial-sized box fans rattle through our tiny apartment, sending powerful gusts of wind against the soggy carpet covering half of the living room. A terrible ice storm blew through our city the week prior, and now the warming spring temperatures have caused the ice to melt so rapidly that it spills over the rain gutters and streams down the walls of our top-floor apartment, soaking the drywall and gathering into carpet pools next to our hand-me-down couch.

Through the wind and noise of those giant fans, I thumb through the book in my hands, *How Al-Anon Works for Families & Friends of Alcoholics*. I should probably focus on my notes from anatomy or study the latest chapter from *Robins Pathologic Basis of Disease*. But I am looking for answers to my main problem: My husband is an addict and won't (actually can't) stop using drugs, my marriage is ending, and my life feels totally out of my control.

At twenty-four years old, I believe that if I can just get my husband to stop drinking and using drugs, if I can just finish up medical school and move into our first house and begin our little family, if I can just get started on my *real* life, then all will be well. And maybe then I can relax my shoulders and feel more fully alive.

I've spent a lifetime hiding behind my accomplishments and attempting to prove my worth, chasing an impossible life plan toward perfection. And now if I can just get a handle on my husband and our marriage, then surely, I won't wonder so often who I am, where I'm going, and what is the point. But in this moment, there is no hiding from myself. My high school sweetheart and now husband of two years is away for a thirty-day stay in drug rehab. My apartment is filled with carpet pools. And I am all alone. The sound of failure reverberates through my ears as those box fans demand, *What now? What now? What are you going to do now?*

I desperately clutch at a solution.

I hope the book in my hands will tell me something I can *do* about this mess. Something I can *do* to fix my husband and our crumbling marriage. But instead, rather annoyingly, it suggests I let go. It tells me to "Keep It Simple" and take "First Things First." It asks me questions like, "How Important Is It?" It proposes that I "Keep an Open Mind" and "Let Go and Let God."[1] This book provides zero suggestions for fixing my husband and no insight into how I can finally achieve the life I long for. And I need answers.

I look up from its pages, and my eyes land on the baby crib I bought on clearance a few weeks prior, now stacked in pieces against the wall of our bedroom waiting for our "someday soon" baby. I burst into laughter through my tears. This isn't an ideal time to start a family, I know. But I have spent my entire life attempting to push my way through, and babies are next on my to-do list. A baby in the middle of medical school with a man who is endlessly hooked on drugs? I know how ridiculous this sounds, but it is the only thing I can think of to *do*.

❋ ❋ ❋ ❋

We believe there must be some secret to happiness, don't we? Some magic trick to creating a happy marriage and a happy family and a happy life, something everyone else knows that we haven't quite figured out. And when we find ourselves floundering through a very real and complicated life that almost never looks as bright and shiny as we hoped, we attempt to overcome our obvious lack of, well . . . *everything* . . . with determination, love, prayer, hard work, meddling, self-help books, perseverance, and pretending. The fancy word for all of it is *control*.

We clamp our fists around our lives and our circumstances and our people, and we attempt to make them bright and shiny. We force ourselves to be happy. We try to strong-arm our way through life. But despite our best efforts, we continue to struggle. And we continue to lose. We hoist more and more onto the heavy load we carry on our backs, trying to do it *all*, attempting to at least pretend to have everything together. Until finally, we grow weary of pretending.

At twenty-four and freshly married, I would need a very long time (a decade, really) to grow weary of pretending. And a few weeks after those carpet pools dried out, when I visited my husband over a long weekend in his drug rehab facility, that's exactly what I did. I pretended. I wore makeup and curled my hair. I tried to coax my drug-addicted husband back into the perfect life I had planned for us. And I set out to convince the others at the rehab facility that he didn't belong there with my overly sure attitude and put-together appearance. I offered hugs and held hands and prayed the prayers. I was the model student in group therapy.

"Oh, yes. It's fine. I'm fine. Yes, I'm learning so much!" *But, also, we don't really belong here.* I was confident in that. After all, several of my husband's peers were missing teeth.

The next few years of worsening drug use and growing debt and aching sadness proved that yes, we absolutely belonged there. It was as heartbreaking to watch as it was impossible to fix; there was just no stopping my husband's steady deterioration. I know because I tried it all.

Then finally one day, during my husband's second stay in rehab (which would be followed by a six-month stay in a three-quarter-way addiction recovery house while I single-parented our two little boys at home), I sat next to the counselor of our therapy group and accidentally told him I was pissed. Seething. Filled with blind, hot rage. My husband was ruining *everything*. He was ruining my perfect life plan. He was ruining both our lives and inadvertently hurting our children with his pain and lies. To me, he was weak and small. And worse, he made me feel fragile and helpless, which was my least favorite thing. I had lived my entire life trying to convince others that I was strong, intelligent, capable, and confident. I was an over-producing, over-achieving, over-working, people-pleasing machine able to crank out more and more and more while promising, *I won't let you down! See? I'm wearing a midriff!* But my husband was blowing my cover. And I could no longer pretend.

I was powerless.

The counselor smiled wide at my young, naïve rage. His face filled with pride as he said gently, "Mikala, look at you! You're *feeling*." And I hated him for it. I did not want to *feel*, I wanted something I could *do*.

But there was nothing to be done.

Sitting with the counselor in that circle of other hurting and lonely people is where I learned there is a truth about me and about this life, something different than what anyone can see from the outside, something broken and real and beloved and beautifully fragile. Of course, I still desperately wanted to prove I was strong, intelligent, capable, and confident. But in those rooms, I was exposed for what I really was—strong *and* incredibly tired, intelligent *and* desperately lonely, capable *and* tragically flawed, beautiful *and* so very afraid.

The "control" I had over my marriage and my plans and my life had only ever been an illusion. That stupid book had been right all along. The question became not "What do I do?" but instead

"What *can* I do?" And when I finally stopped pretending, the answer became clear: *I am the only person I can change.*

My change began with radical acceptance. I had to accept what was true. Accept that the man I loved was hooked on drugs and alcohol. Accept that he had lied to me repeatedly. Accept that his actions had hurt me deeply in a way that was possibly beyond repair. Accept that the whole experience had peeled away a shiny exterior layer of my life, exposing a raw nerve underneath, and that pain and sorrow and loss are part of a good, hard, ordinary life. Accept that hard—even excruciating—feelings are a normal reaction to painful experiences and that focusing on myself would surely lead to more pain as I began to reveal the truth of who I really am. Accept that I might become a single mom and the solo breadwinner for our two little boys. Accept that what zapped at my heart like the unbearable, exposed-nerve pain of loss now would surely sting less eventually if I took it one day at a time.

The Serenity Prayer became an extremely powerful tool to moving bravely forward through my life and finding a place of comfort. And even all these years later (when I remember to stop pretending) I continue to rely on God to sort out what I can and cannot *do*.

> God, grant me the serenity
> To accept the things I cannot change,
> Courage to change the things I can,
> And wisdom to know the difference.[2]
>
> Reinhold Niebuhr

The beautiful truth of the Serenity Prayer is universal to every single person on the planet and relevant to all areas of our lives—relationships, career, parenting and children, our changing health, love, and the inevitabilities of a very real and complicated life. Turns out, our greatest source of pain will always be our own continued attempt to control and change the people and events in our lives over which we are completely powerless because there is nothing we can actually do to change what is horribly true. The Serenity Prayer suggests a better way. Instead of constantly wrestling for control, we can first seek to find acceptance, bearing witness to the true, hard facts of our lives before finding the courage to change what we can. And remembering, always, to ask God for the wisdom to know the difference.

- God, when and where do I act?
- God, when and how do I let go?
- And God, why? Why does life and love and living and growing old in this place with the people we hold so dear have to be so incredibly hard?

I wonder if we will ever stop asking why.

When it comes to our health, the "beauty and wellness" industry and America's consumer culture insist there *is* an answer to controlling and fixing both our bodies and our lives—a new anti-aging solution, the next all "natural" supplement for perfect health, some no-fail organizational system or eating plan or exercise program. We are surrounded by incessant messaging that repeatedly promises: *You can be thinner! You can be eternally young and smooth! You can be fit and healthy and toned and free of pain or chronic illness and not to mention perfect and successful and so ridiculously happy! This goes for your family, too, because YOU are in control!*

But the painful reality is, we can't achieve the impossible in our bodies, in our relationships, or in our lives. And we are driving ourselves (and probably our loved ones) to insanity by exerting our power and influence to force a certain outcome into being. Instead, the only thing to do when life shatters to the floor is to take everything apart piece by piece, then hold the broken bits up to the light and examine them—asking, *Is this piece mine? Do I need this? Is this important? Or necessary? Can I let this go? Should I let this go? To find serenity, do I need to let this go?*

Digging Deeper into "the Control Filter"

It's maddening that we can't control our lives, isn't it? I know. It feels nearly impossible sometimes to embrace that this is true. But it is important to acknowledge that in any situation, we can only control what we can control. And for all the rest? Acceptance is a good option. Letting go, accepting the results, and beginning to control only what we *can* control is a transformative experience that will truly change your life.

When we are hit with a crisis, we can begin to sift. We can keep only what matters and shake away the rest, hoping to clear a path back to wholeness using the Serenity Prayer for answers. We can examine each situation and relationship and hardship in our lives through the filter of control using the following questions:

- Which parts of my life are mine to control or possibly change?
- And which are not?
- Which pieces of this current situation can I do anything about?
- And where do I need to let go?
- What choices are mine to make?
- God, will you point me toward the ways I can change for the better and make the best decisions for *my* life and the body I *actually* have? And God, will you help me to let go of the rest?

There is much to be learned from pain. Namely, that life *will* go on even if you do not get what you want. Bills will come due. Grass will need to be mowed. You will be hungry or tired or bored. You'll use the bathroom and take showers and occasionally walk a full bag of garbage out to the trash. On your drive to work, another driver will smile from her little red Volvo and wave you into traffic, making room.

The world will keep turning, and you'll wonder how. *How?*

How are people selecting ripe pears from the stack at the store and tying up those little plastic bags before gently placing them in the cart? How are they filling their cars with gas or circling through the drive-thru for coffee? Why are they laughing? What can possibly be so funny when the whole world has . . . stopped?

It's easy to forget that we're human, isn't it?

Sometimes we get irritated at the slow checkout line lady or annoyed when the barista gets our order wrong in the drive-thru. We grumble about lawyers or overpriced HVAC repairmen. We say things like, "Those damn doctors!"

But we're *all* human. And we never really know what another person is going through. Perhaps that barista's mother is dying a slow, debilitating death from Alzheimer's disease or her child is struggling with dyslexia and ADHD and yesterday was a very messy IEP meeting with the school. Or perhaps that damn doctor's husband has just left for drug rehab and she's single-parenting two little boys at home. Though the rest of the world keeps moving, keeps driving, keeps shuffling through the grocery store or swinging through Starbucks, today it feels like one person's world is ending. We are *all* suffering from this human condition, and sometimes the pain of it hurts like hell.

Of course, if you'd had a baby, a neighbor might bring dinner to help lighten your load. Family might call to check in, *How are you? Are you getting any rest?* But as it is, no one knows quite what to do when you're struggling with a chronic but invisible disease or you're the single caregiver to aging parents or your mother can't remember your name due to the effects of Alzheimer's disease. And it turns out, no one brings a casserole when your husband goes to rehab. The world just . . . moves on, even when your life has come to a screeching halt from whatever painful, unimaginable thing has just taken your breath away.

Mostly people do not know about your silent pain (possibly because you continue smiling and showing up to work and curling your hair or wearing midriffs then circling through the drive-thru and assuring everyone you are fine). So, they just keep moving, keep smiling, keep living. It doesn't seem fair. I know.

But, somehow, eventually, and probably due to a lack of other options, *you* will too. You will stop pretending, loosen your grip, and eventually move through the pain. You'll let it pierce your heart, and instead of falling over dead from grief, you'll be shocked to find yourself still standing. You'll shop for groceries and push your cart up and down the aisles and pluck a few ripe pears from the stack. You'll make appointments and call the plumber and pay the bills and mow the grass. You'll paint a wall in your house the perfect shade of blue, and you'll be surprised when it makes you smile. You'll go to church and show up for work and laugh at stupid reality TV shows. You'll wonder if it's even okay to laugh when your world is so broken. *Is it really okay to feel happy?* Then you'll occasionally go out for lunch with a friend.

At first, you will feel like an empty shell. Just a ghostly version of yourself going through the motions of this ridiculous life because your heart lies broken and shattered on the floor. You will wonder how you can possibly get through it. *Another day? And then another? Again, how?* And over and over, you'll hit your knees and pray the Serenity Prayer. You'll slip on the Control Filter and begin to make small changes over which you have some level of control. You'll begin to pick up the pieces of your shattered heart from the floor and tuck them safely into your pocket. And you'll pray for something, anything, to change.

Focus on Healing

You must sift. You must begin to realize some parts of life are very important and deserve your time and effort and attention, and others are just the bits of white fluff that have mostly wasted your time. You must decide to let all the excess fall away, keeping only the very important parts. And, slowly, incrementally, bit by bit *you* will change. You will learn to control only those things you can control and practice letting go of (and healing from) the rest.

Embracing the bitter and the sweet, and then learning to let go completely, is a crucial part of midlife. And looking at life through the Control Filter is a tactic we must practice *forever*.

To help, I've compiled a list of all the things you can control

- Your words
- Your attitudes and opinions
- Your thoughts
- Your actions and reactions
- Your choices in life moving forward
- How you spend your time and attention

I suppose what I'm talking about here is **agency,** which is our ability to own and control our own thoughts and actions. Did you notice what *isn't* included on the list? Your background, your history, your upbringing, your socioeconomic barriers, our culture's underlying discriminations, your genetics, your previous traumas, your DNA, and many of the things that do in fact pertain to *you* and your body and your one precious, beautiful life but remain largely out of your control. Yes, you do have agency over your body and yourself, but often your ingrained reactions and emotions, your thoughts, and your behaviors are largely due to outside circumstances that have conspired together to form patterns without you even realizing it.[3]

What we need to harness here instead is our *limited* **agency,** or our ability to recognize destructive patterns and grasp control of those things over which we *actually* have some influence. We can then begin to make changes with our words and attitudes, our reactions, and our choices. With limited agency we can keep the focus on controlling ourselves and relax our grip on all the things that will always remain out of our reach.[4]

So here, I've also provided an exhaustive list of all the things you can't control

- Everything (and everyone) else

It was forever ago, and yesterday. But during those seven years married to my husband while he was actively using drugs, his vacant eyes and trembly hands made it increasingly clear to me that he was gone—lost and wandering through his life and very likely going to die from his addiction. I had exhausted *every possible thing* I could think of to bring him back—back to me and our lives, back to our children, back to light and sobriety and life. But none of it worked. "Fixing" him was out of my control, and I had to let go. I had to let go of trying. I had to relax my grip. I had to sift. And after years of pain and heartbreak and sadness and devastation, two trips to rehab, a six-month stay in a three-quarter-way addiction recovery house, and approximately one million minutes unclenching my fists, I did. *I let him go.*

I harnessed my limited agency, and I learned to do the next right thing. And then the next. And the next. I bought pears from the store. I mowed the lawn. I painted my walls the perfect shade of blue, and it made me smile. I prayed the Serenity Prayer. And every day—every moment, really—I let go. Because in life, *I* am the only person I can control.

Today I have a marriage of twenty-two years to my husband, who has been in recovery now for fifteen years. I have five children and a career and extended family and neighbors and friendships. And I am *still* learning to look at my life through the lens of control. Each day, it feels like I have a whole new list of bits and pieces and broken parts that I pull from my pocket to hold up to the light and question, *Is this mine?* And each day I pray for serenity and acceptance, for the courage to act on my own behalf, and for wisdom to know which parts of life are *mine* to change. I am still practicing the fine art of letting the excess fall away.

One of the most important discoveries of midlife is learning to peel your fingers back from the death grip you've had on relationships, health, kids, career, life, and the picture you've carried in your mind for so long of how life is *supposed* to be. I'm sorry. I know it hurts, but it doesn't look the way you hoped. And no matter how hard you struggle and fight, it just isn't going to be that way. But it *can* be beautiful in a whole new way if you can only let go of control.

When we learn to look through the Control Filter, when we learn to sift, we just may find serenity. Now (or for at least five minutes every day) I have found mine. It takes a lifetime of practice but, my dear friend, *you* are the only person you can change.

5

"WE CAN DO ANY(*EVERY*)THING" AND ADULT ATTENTION DEFICIT HYPERACTIVITY DISORDER

I am sitting outside a conference room before my interview for medical school in a camel-colored suit with a bright blue shirt peeking over the jacket collar. I'm hoping this unique color might set me apart from the sea of navy and gray suits on my peers.

I feel well prepared for every possible question and come ready to discuss my hard work ethic and achievements during under-grad, my empathetic nature and easy way with people, my long résumé of volunteer opportunities, my love of science, and my in-tentions to pursue family medicine or pediatrics during residency. I've planned for this moment for four grueling years of college and recently completed the seven-hour medical college admission test (MCAT) with an admirable, above average score.

As I wait for my turn, I think back to the evening my mother cornered me in the kitchen after parent-teacher conferences in high school and said, "Did you know you're ranked first in your class?"

At the time I didn't realize anyone was keeping track, so I shrugged and continued unloading dishes from the dishwasher.

She went on with a mixture of pride and knowing in her voice, "Your counselor says you could study just about anything you want in college, and Dad and I think you should be a pediatrician! Wouldn't that be fun? Taking care of all those babies?"

My dad mumbled something from the couch in the other room about "golfing in the afternoons, too," and my mother returned to peeling potatoes for our stew. I let my mind wander as I divided forks and knives and spoons into the drawer. *First in the class, huh?* Medical school did seem like a pretty good idea. After all, I loved kids. And science. Plus, it all came with a fancy title.

It would take only four years for a bachelor of science degree, four years of medical school for a doctorate, plus three more easy-peasy years in residency, then BOOM! I'd have my big salary for doing a respectable career so I could live in a fancy house with my perfect family taking care of babies and golfing in the afternoon (though, in truth, I had absolutely no desire to golf). Maybe that *was* the answer to what I should do with my life. By the time we sat down to dinner that evening, the matter was settled. I had a plan. And I had no reason to question whether I could do it all. Of course I could!

Anything. Anything you want. A woman can do anything.

Six years later, with a bachelor of science degree (with honors, no less) alongside an impressive résumé and the sheer determination to succeed, it is suddenly my turn. I stand and confidently smooth the front of my camel-colored suit before I enter the conference room and sit down. After a very brief introduction, the man conducting my interview looks up from my paperwork and peers at me for a moment over his reading glasses. Then he asks, "Are you married?"

"Yes?" I ask, suddenly feeling unsure.

"What will you do when your child is home sick, but you are on call at the hospital with a clinic full of patients to see? What will you do when your sick child wants his mother?"

I am not prepared for this question. I never saw this particular question on the list of "How to Prepare for Your Medical School Interview." My face grows hot and my body tingles with a mixture of embarrassment and rage as I stammer something about how lucky I am to have parents living nearby who would probably be willing to help. Then I leave the interview feeling bewildered and . . . well . . . furious. My mind races. *Would he ask that question of the other candidates? The candidates in the gray and navy suits? The male candidates? After all, a woman can do anything a man can do. Anything. And who says a woman's place is at home with a sick child? Of course I'll be able to do it all! And what about this sick, hypothetical child's father? Where was he?*

My family life feels like none of my interviewer's business, and I simply cannot believe the audacity of this man to ask how I might balance my home life as a wife and a mom with the rigorous demands of practicing medicine. Weeks later, when I receive my acceptance letter, I set out to prove him wrong—I will be an amazing mother *and* a doctor; I will somehow manage to be on call overnight at the hospital *and* at home raising my children. I will be absolutely everything anyone ever needs me to be because I am a feminist.[1] I am strong and intelligent and capable and worthy. I can do anything a man can do, and more.

Anything. Anything I want. A woman can do anything.

This was the messaging of the women's movement, right? A woman can do *anything.* My first semester in medical school at the Nebraska Medical Center in Omaha was the first year in university history that the number of men to women entering medicine was split evenly, 50/50. It felt important to me somehow. *Women can do anything! See?* We're creative, capable, intelligent, hardworking, kindhearted, and strong. We bring incredible value to our families and our workplaces and our communities. Women can absolutely change the world. I believe that with all my heart. But for me, and for many women, something about this empowering messaging got lost in translation. Somehow, instead of liberating us from a small, tidy box and a "woman's place," the world silently and maliciously altered the narrative: *You want to be a feminist, huh? Okay, that's great. But to be a strong and capable and worthy woman and exist as an "equal" in this sphere, you need to do the work of both a man AND a woman. You need to do it ALL.*

Of course, we long to be strong and capable and worthy. We want to exist in this sphere. So, we knock ourselves out trying to bring home the bacon *and* fry it up in the pan. We fill our schedules and take fitness classes and volunteer at the kids' school and follow five-year plans to success. We are dependable, on time, overly prepared, selfless, and constantly moving. If asked, we are fine. More than fine. We are amazing!

We live in a generation of women empowered to do anything we put our minds to! Except most of us were also raised with traditional gender roles, so somehow we are still the primary caregivers and nurturers of our beautiful and loving homes. And many of us wholeheartedly believe what the world continues to sell us: *This is what it means to be a strong woman—the only way to BE enough is to DO enough.* So, we mostly try to stay out of everyone's way and remain agreeable while also believing we can (and should!) do *every single thing* the world demands:

- Work a full-time job with a lucrative salary
- Manage a perfect household
- Keep an impeccably clean, organized, and beautifully decorated home
- Contribute to our neighborhoods and churches in creative and exciting ways
- Spearhead ministry work and volunteering
- Remember to practice that all-important "self-care" (i.e., maintain a smokin' hot bod for regular sex with our spouse)
- Be productive outside of motherhood while simultaneously raising perfect prodigy children as the primary caregiver and nurturer of a loving home

- Succeed at basically everything everywhere while also managing to care for a sick child at home who wants his mother
- And do it *all* without help or support

We give and we give and we give, then we feel guilty if we ever dare to take in return. We somehow forget to treat *ourselves* the way we treat others and allow self-criticism and martyrdom to beat a rhythm on the drums to which we tirelessly dance—around and around and around—hoping to prove our worth.

Turns out, we completely misheard the feminists before us who claimed the authority and gathered the accolades and shouted with encouragement and pride to every woman following behind, "Women can do anything!" And we've taken to heart the faulty idea that *women should be EVERYthing*. Then, when we grow tired and weary and inevitably fail at the unachievable expectations the world has set for us, we wonder quietly . . . *Hmmm, do I have adult ADHD???*

I personally spent years (decades, really) shouting, "I am strong and intelligent and capable and worthy! I am a feminist! I can do *anything*! No, even better, I can do *every*thing! See? I am worthy! I can do it ALL!" while thinking inwardly, *I mean, I guess. Maybe I can do it all. Wait. Can anyone really do it all?* But my success made everyone around me so happy that I couldn't stop striving. I desperately wanted to prove my worth—I wanted to exist in this sphere—but I simply could not win at what is obviously a rigged game. And I completely exhausted myself trying.

❋ ❋ ❋ ❋

I had been working in private practice for four years while raising three little boys at home and repairing a marriage scarred by addiction, when one evening my now sober husband looked up from his computer with a glimmer of excitement in his eyes, "What

79

do you think about Utah?" He was soon to finish his training in pathology and needed to apply for his final fellowship year.

My mind raced. *I don't know. What's in Utah? What about my work? What about this career I've been building for a decade? And what about our family, my parents, my friends, all our activities? What will we tell them? Can we just . . . leave? How exactly do I upend this life I've been trying to stuff myself into for years?*

Our move one thousand miles away to the mountains of Utah felt like ripping my "successful" life at the seams. As we pulled away from the curb, our boys' neighborhood friends, who spent most summer afternoons playing in the blow-up pool in our side yard laughing or fighting like siblings and stopping only for popsicles, ran along behind the moving van for as long as they could keep up, waving and crying. My children were crying in the backseat. And I hesitated. *Wait, where are we going? Why are we doing this? What's in Utah again?*

But then I remembered the feeling of relief that washed over me when I returned the hospital pager I'd been carrying on my hip for so many years. It felt like handing over a giant lead weight. An anvil. A cement block tied to my feet that I'd been kicking against for years, flailing and treading while trying desperately to keep my face above water. I had been jolted with electrical shocks of anxiety from one pager or another for almost a decade as if I had a taser strapped to my waistline, each time giving me heart palpitations and a little zinger of adrenaline. I can still, after all this time, recall the exact chirp in my mind, alerting me of something I needed to *do.* Immediately. Any memory of that pager still brings a tiny wave of nausea. Doo doo dee doo dooop. Doo doo dee doo dooop.

But I would never carry a pager again. *I don't work there anymore.*

The truth beneath all those accolades and all that striving was that I had been wearing my life like a shirt that was too tight. It *looked* okay, I guess. It zipped up in back and matched my dress slacks and cardigan, and on the outside, I appeared to be "put

80

together." My husband was three years clean and sober after a treacherous time in medical school and residency and several trips to visit him in drug rehab. I worked three long days a week between the clinic and hospital while my parents watched our boys, who were seven, five, and two. The older boys enjoyed basketball and soccer through our local YMCA on weekends. We drove a used minivan. And our oldest, Isaiah, thrived in first grade at the public school in our neighborhood. On the weekends, I ran half marathons and participated in book clubs and Bible studies and decorated our cookie-cutter home with half-priced finds from Home Goods. Then every week, I went to Al-Anon meetings on Sundays after church. And life was . . . fine. Good. Successful, even.

But sometimes if I breathed in too deep or too wide, I felt like I might burst. I moved frantically through my days taking shallow breaths and sucking in my stomach and trying to smile and appear calm, collected, and successful without ever fully breathing. I was managing it! I was a strong woman! *See?* I was doing it all!

Still, at the end of every day, I could barely wriggle myself out of a life that felt too tight. I had to flip my head over and attempt to pull everything I was carrying up over my shoulders with both arms, wiggling and sweating like when I panic in the dressing room wondering if I'll have to ask the salesperson to grab some scissors and cut me free of a shirt that is one size too small. Every day I attempted to shrink myself to fit while muttering expletives through the sound of tiny micro-rips that warned, *It's too much. It's too tight!* The life I had been living just never really . . . fit.

When we packed up and moved to Utah, I left so much of my life behind. I left the state I grew up in, my college girlfriends, a neighborhood full of other moms my age and my kids' little friends. I left my budding career doing both outpatient clinic and inpatient hospital medicine just miles from the same medical institution where I had trained for seven years. I left my children's extracurricular activities, my sister and her children, my parents' home only a five-minute drive up the road, my book club and half marathons and Bible study. It felt terrible. But also, for the first time in a very long time I felt like I could exhale and breeeeaaaaathe. I had finally wriggled myself free.

It turns out, women can do many, many things (truly just about anything we put our minds to), but despite the messaging we hear from the world that we must do more and more and more to prove our value and worth, we simply cannot do *every*thing—especially without support.

It makes me wonder about the load you've been carrying . . .

- Have you been listening to the demands of the world and the endless expectations of women, attempting to do it *all*?
- Are your days filled with tightly packed schedules and 5:00 a.m. yoga and emails from the teacher and seemingly endless meetings at work and a running grocery list and your kid's turn for soccer treats and orthodontist appointments (again) and helping your aging mother on Saturday and college application paperwork with your teen and therapy appointments and a never-ending list of to-dos around the house?
- When you inevitably fall short and begin dropping balls or silently longing to free yourself from a life that feels too tight, do you sometimes wonder if it's just . . . you? Do you think to yourself, *Is there something wrong with me? Are other people better at keeping it all together? Is it just . . . me?*
- Do you wonder if you might be missing an underlying problem that explains your repeated forgetfulness or those frequently missed deadlines or your inability to finish tasks or why you can't seem to complete a single thought?
- Is this a result of adult ADHD or are you simply attempting to carry too much?

Many of us struggle with the unreasonable expectations of the world and the incessant barrage of incoming stimuli via news and movies and YouTube videos and side conversations with other moms at the park and never-ending social media posts. In this modern age, our brains are forced to process exponentially more information than ever before, and then we wonder about a diagnosis of adult ADHD because we don't feel motivated or productive, we can't stay focused on one task, we can't ever seem to get anything accomplished, and sometimes we walk into a room and can't remember why we walked in there.

The expectations placed on women today are, in short, ridiculous. Not only that, but we also have immediate access to endless information (both vital and frivolous). Our brains have had to develop new habits to cope and process it all, often leaving us feeling unfocused, scatterbrained, and forgetful. In their book *ADHD 2.0: New Science and Essential Strategies for Thriving with Distraction—from Childhood through Adulthood*, Drs. Hallowell and Ratey describe the term for this phenomenon as **VAST, or variable attention stimulus trait,** which they describe as an "environmentally induced cousin" of ADHD.[2]

Women universally relate to feeling overwhelmed by the stuff of life and the invisible emotional labor of being a woman, but *the extent to which our overwhelm impairs our functioning* is the difference between having an official diagnosis of ADHD or not. So, how exactly do we decipher between simply having too much on our plates (i.e., attempting to do any(*every*)thing the world throws our way) and an underlying medical condition like adult ADHD?

Digging Deeper into Adult ADHD

ADHD, like most neurodivergent diagnoses, exists on a spectrum. Often discovered during childhood due to "problem" behavior in school, disorganization, inability to complete tasks, frequent interruptions during classroom discussions, and a general lack of functioning to a child's full "potential," it was once believed that children can outgrow ADHD. We understand now that ADHD almost universally persists into adulthood, and those adults who seem to have outgrown their childhood ADHD have simply learned to compensate so well that their symptoms largely disappear.

For those who receive a formal diagnosis of ADHD in adulthood, many symptoms of ADHD were likely present since childhood; however, such symptoms may only become blatantly obvious once the demands of busy (often overwhelming) adult life exceed the ability to counterbalance the deficits. Examples include when a college student heads off to graduate school, when a woman becomes a mom, when a mid-level employee receives a promotion and takes on a management position, or when a woman finds herself firmly in the "sandwich" role, taking care of her own children and family as well as her aging parents. Suddenly in this new high-demand role, the requirements for organizational skills and attention to detail increase dramatically, which overwhelms the **cognitive load** (the amount our brains can process at any one time)[3] and results in upheaval in work or life.

But how can we tell if it's ADHD?

The ADHD brain in adulthood tends to be "here, there, and everywhere." And without intervention and ongoing support, missed deadlines, forgotten obligations, and lost opportunities (oh, and almost daily lost car keys) may frequently result. Managing time can be a challenge, and running behind becomes commonplace. In addition, those with ADHD may have a low tolerance for stress and feel extremely sensitive to criticism, working tirelessly to conform to the expectations of adult life and often over-committing to responsibilities that can't be fulfilled, which causes incredible internalized shame. Feeling disorganized, scattered, forgetful, easily distracted, flighty, hypersensitive to the environment (the noises, sights, and smells) or just generally "never living up to potential" may all point to a formal ADHD diagnosis.[4]

While almost *all* of us have a ridiculous number of plates we must keep spinning between work, marriage, parenting, caregiver roles, healthy habits, household chores, church or volunteer commitments, and more, those who struggle with symptoms of ADHD without intervention may suffer higher rates of more severe negative consequences such as job loss, criminal activity, broken relationships, substance abuse problems in an attempt to self-medicate, and traffic accidents or tickets compared to adults without an ADHD diagnosis. Early, appropriate, and ongoing interventions, however, can help unleash the *gifts* of the ADHD brain, which often include incredible creativity, ingenuity, empathy and emotional sensitivity, amazing resilience, spontaneity, boundless energy, and a wonderful capacity for joy.

The challenge of making a diagnosis of ADHD is that there isn't blood work or an imaging study to use as a diagnostic tool. Instead, we rely on a list of criteria and evaluate the level of impairment in overall functioning in multiple areas, including both home and work life.

Symptoms of adult ADHD fit into three categories[5]

HYPERACTIVITY SYMPTOMS

- Fidgeting or restlessness
- Talking a lot
- Constant activity
- A tendency to choose extremely active daily jobs

IMPULSIVITY SYMPTOMS

- Abruptly ending relationships
- Interrupting in conversations or difficulty with verbal processing
- Quitting jobs frequently
- Overreacting to frustrating events
- Accumulating traffic citations and accidents

INATTENTION SYMPTOMS

- Procrastination
- Trouble listening

- Difficulty making decisions
- Poor time management and attention
- Forgetfulness or losing things frequently
- Difficulty in organizing or completing tasks
- Distractibility
- Anxiety and low self-esteem

For kiddos, we evaluate ADHD symptoms using a bunch of questionnaires answered by both parents and teachers to assess the severity of a child's symptoms and any resulting difficulties they may experience in *multiple* settings. For adults, however, the severity of symptoms is typically evaluated through self-report, and it can look a little different for everyone.[6] I've included a screening tool on the following page, which is helpful for recognizing the warning signs of ADHD and may indicate a need for further evaluation by your medical provider.[7]

If an at-home screening test for ADHD is positive, it's important to have a discussion with your primary provider and complete a more in-depth rating scale like the Conners' Adult ADHD Rating Scale or the Adult ADHD Self-Report Scale. An ADHD exam with a doctor will also exclude any other possible diagnoses like thyroid disease or an underlying mood disorder using blood work and more extensive questioning/questionnaires.

There's something called the "big book of psychiatric disorders" titled the **Diagnostic and Statistical Manual of Mental Disorders (DSM-5-TR)**, which provides the official diagnostic criteria for adult ADHD.[8]

Diagnostic criteria for adult ADHD

- Five or more symptoms are present from either the inattention or impulsivity categories
- Symptoms must be present for six months or more without another explanation (such as depression, anxiety, or another contributing factor)

Adult ADHD Screening Tool

The following questionnaire can be used as a starting point to help recognize the signs/symptoms of adult ADHD but is not meant to replace consultation with a trained healthcare professional. An accurate diagnosis can only be made through a clinical evaluation.

This Adult Self-Report Scale—V1.1 (ASRA-V1.1) Screener is intended for people age 18 years or older.

Check the box that best describes how you have felt and conducted yourself over the past 6 months.	Never	Rarely	Sometimes	Often	Very Often
1. How often do you have trouble wrapping up the final details of a project once the challenging parts have been done?					
2. How often do you have difficulty getting things in order when you have to do a task that requires organization?					
3. How often do you have problems remembering appointments or obligations?					
4. When you have a task that requires a lot of thought, how often do you avoid or delay getting started?					
5. How often do you fidget or squirm with your hands or feet when you have to sit down for a long time?					
6. How often do you feel overly active and compelled to do things, like you were driven by a motor?					

GRADING: Add the number of checkmarks that appear in the darkly shaded areas. Four or more checkmarks indicate that your symptoms may be consistent with adult ADHD. It may be beneficial for you to talk with your family physician about an evaluation.

- AND several symptoms have to have been present since age twelve
- Symptoms must be present in at least two settings and cause a limitation in social, occupational, or academic functioning

ADHD can be predominantly inattentive, predominantly hyperactive, or have a combined presentation. Symptoms are rated from mild to moderate or severe and can morph or change in form or severity over time. We often begin treatment by focusing on skill-building and making adaptations for time management, organization, and planning. For some, these adaptive skills developed through lifestyle changes are not enough, and improved attention comes through a combination of environmental modifications *and* stimulant medications like amphetamines or methylphenidate (or atomoxetine or bupropion for those who can't tolerate the side effects such as dry mouth, poor sleep, irritability, headaches, or decreased appetite that can occur from taking a stimulant).[9]

If you screened positively on the above tool, you may feel the most comfortable talking with a psychiatrist or therapist specifically trained in adult ADHD, especially if you and your medical provider feel that treatment with medication is warranted.

Focus on Healing

The ADHD brain repeatedly shifts your attention to here and here and here and here, making it difficult to remain focused and complete your day-to-day tasks, kind of like this quote from Iain Thomas:

> And every day, the world [insert ADHD] will drag you by the hand, yelling, "This is important! And this is important! And this is important! You need to worry about this! And this! And this!" And each day, it's up to you to yank your hand back, put it on your heart and say, "No. This is what's important."[10]

It may be a challenge, but you *can* put systems in place to limit distractions, train your brain for improved concentration, and harness all the big, beautiful creativity that comes along with ADHD to create something necessary, productive, and wonderful with your life.

Many of the adaptive skills used for treatment of adult ADHD are beneficial for *any* woman who is struggling in her attempt to do *every*thing (and perhaps suffering from the stimulation overload of VAST as we discussed above) with or without a formal adult ADHD diagnosis.

Helpful day-to-day adjustments for improved focus and organization

1. **Create daily routines (morning, lunch, after school/work, evening, bedtime)** and a general flow or *schedule* to follow throughout your day. For an adult with ADHD, structure is your friend. But please remember to keep it simple. *Too* rigid a structure may lead to poor follow-through. Some people benefit from a simple color-coded paper calendar while others prefer to use one or two daily alarms (because any more than this just becomes extra noise) to help keep them on track.

2. **Evaluate where you are doing too much.** Take some time to look at your daily/weekly/monthly activities and offload something (or many things). Slip on the Control Filter we talked about in chapter 4 and begin looking around at your life—where can you let go? Can you delegate a few things? Can you give a firm NO to something else? Where can you simplify your schedule? Where can you ask for or hire more support? It's time to eliminate extra friction in your life. I know you're carrying way too much!

3. **Do a weekly brain dump.** On the same day every week (try Sunday evening or Monday morning), write down everything you've been ruminating on lately. Get it all out and down on paper so it can stop replaying on a loop in your mind. Then, choose only *three* to-dos from the weekly brain dump and put them onto each day's list. Any more than that can be overwhelming and prevent you from completing a single thing on the list.

4. **Practice *single* tasking.** Rather than listening to a podcast while running the vacuum or talking on the phone to a

friend while uploading that file at work, quiet the noise and practice doing only *one thing at a time*.

5. **Declutter your life.** Create a safe and happy haven for your brain to learn and work in by eliminating unnecessary clutter from your environment. Our brains are heavily influenced by our surroundings, and it's hard to concentrate with stuff everywhere. Clean out your purse and your car. Ruthlessly declutter your home and your wardrobe. Organize your desk at work. Invest the time and energy *now* to sift through your belongings and give your brain a clean and streamlined state to be productive in.

6. **Eat a healthy diet.** This one is a must for ADHD! In general, healthy eating includes whole foods with fruits and vegetables, lean protein, healthy fats, and plenty of water. Avoid processed foods, sugar, and caffeine whenever possible since too much of these foods can worsen the symptoms of ADHD.

7. **Limit (or completely avoid) screen time.** Some experts recommend no more than two hours of screen time per day. You can begin by regularly turning off your device or putting it aside for at least several hours every day, especially when you are trying to focus your attention on another project. And at night, be sure to store your phone in another room away from where you sleep and opt not to have a TV, tablet, or other device in your bedroom.

8. **Exercise regularly.** One role of both stimulants and antidepressants prescribed for ADHD is to increase dopamine, serotonin, and norepinephrine in the brain. Exercise can do this, too! Getting regular daily exercise through aerobic activity, strength training, and flexibility/balance techniques increases arousal and attention, especially for those with ADHD. Simply find something you enjoy!

After all, the best kind of exercise is the exercise you will actually *do*.

9. **Ask for help.** Children with an ADHD diagnosis generally have an IEP to improve accommodations and services for learning in the classroom. Consider creating your own individualized life program (let's call it an ILP) to optimize your full potential at work, at home, and in all areas of your life. You will likely need help from your medical provider for medications or referrals, from a therapist or social coach who can assist you with schedules and routines, from your coworkers or boss for necessary accommodations at work, and from your close friends and family members to help with adjustments at home and offer support in your day-to-day activities.

10. **Prioritize rest and sleep.** Because ADHD is linked to overactivity, it is especially necessary to pay attention to sleep. Try to get seven to eight hours of good-quality sleep each night. We'll talk more about sleep, sleep disorders, and the importance of bedroom hygiene in chapter 10.

The response of ADHD symptoms to treatment with lifestyle modifications, ongoing support, and prescription medication is monitored by a self-report ADHD symptom checklist combined with objective information such as job performance evaluations, attendance records, grades, or promotions.

I do not have an adult ADHD diagnosis; however, I am learning to practice the above adaptations and slowly decrease the unnecessary clutter and noise pulling me in a thousand different directions each day and distracting my attention. Though I still have a million things to attend to every week between our five kids and my work requirements and our crazy schedules and the basic household chores and everyone's needs and our lengthy list of dermatologist/orthodontist/optometry appointments and the grocery shopping and laundry and everything else, today I am living a much quieter life. A beautiful, *ordinary* life.

When we moved to Utah, somehow I managed to slip the Control Filter into so many areas of my existence that I'd not stopped to consider before—my words, my thoughts, my attitudes and opinions, my actions and reactions, my choices, and how I spend my time and attention. I began making thoughtful decisions for my one precious, beautiful life and asking for more support.

Now when people ask why we moved from the familiarity of Nebraska and all our friends and family to the mountains of Utah, I tell them it's because my husband needed to complete a fellowship year to finish up his medical training. I tell them it's because he was offered a great job at the same institution, plus I found a medical group where I could work very, very part-time, maintain my licensure (without a pager), and mostly stay home with our kids. Sometimes I tell them it's because we love the outdoors—the skiing and hiking, the wildflowers and beautiful mountain views. But really, it's because the life I had been attempting to stuff myself into had stopped fitting at all. And when I completely ripped apart at the seams, Utah opened itself to us, welcoming us inside a whole new way of living and being and doing and breathing. A life in which we could move freely, choosing only the things that fit us just right. One where every day I can breathe big and deep and wide, believing I am strong and intelligent and capable and loved regardless of my achievements. *I truly exist in this sphere*, and the comfort of these mountains both streamlined and salvaged my life.

We can do many, many things. It's true. But we do not have to do it *all*.

If you're struggling with focus and follow-through, it might be due to adult ADHD. Or perhaps you are simply juggling too much. You can start by working through the above suggestions, and maybe you'll find improvement without a formal diagnosis. If you need more help, consider talking to your medical provider to discuss medication. Your personal provider is the best source of information for questions and concerns related to your symptoms of adult ADHD or possibilities for treatment. Whatever works best for you, please remember this one very important truth: Women really can do *anything*, but we do not have to do *everything* to prove our worth.

6

RAGE, PREMENSTRUAL DYSPHORIC DISORDER, AND CHANGES OF THE LATER REPRODUCTIVE YEARS

A text came through as I pulled into the car line to pick the kids up from school: *If you have a minute, will you give me a call?* I could tell it was an SOS signal.

So, after we got home and I listened to my children's most pressing details of the day and everyone was settled in with snacks and homework supplies and cartoons, I called back.

"What's going on? Everything okay?" I asked, rocking on the old green glider in the corner of our bedroom.

"Well, my stupid hormones almost got me fired today," came the beloved voice of my dear friend on the other side.

"Really? What happened?"

"I called my boss the B-word. I can't believe I used that word. I hate that word! But I just couldn't take it anymore!"

She paused for a moment and added thoughtfully, "I mean, I wasn't really *wrong*." And we laughed as she filled me in on the rest of the story, lamenting the ridiculousness of our middle-aged, hormonal bodies and emotions.

"So, what happens now?" I asked.

"Oh, I showed up to her office an hour later and apologized. I think I smoothed things over. No surprise I'm about to start my period. I've been walking around yelling at everyone for two days. I've *got* to do something about this. Once a month I feel like I'm going completely crazy, and then three days later I'm fine. I mean, *mostly* fine."

I agreed. It was time to see her doctor.

Unfortunately, I know that rage-y feeling all too well. I know the hot, uncontrollable rush of anger that bursts forth and erupts from my chest, often over something so heinous as a cup of spilled milk. To be fair, sometimes it's the *second* cup of spilled milk for the day, and the milk rolls over the side of the table, splashing onto the floor and soaking our new rug in the kitchen— the blue rug with the rust-colored accents that pulls the whole room together, the one I searched endlessly for online until I found just the right color to match both the paint in the other room and the throw pillows on our couch (on sale from Lowe's, who knew?).

As milk splatters to the rug under the table, everyone sits there blinking back at me, stunned. Unmoving. And the only thing to do as I grab frantically for the paper towels is scream at the top of my lungs, "WHAT ARE YOU DOING? DON'T JUST SIT THERE! DO SOMETHING! THIS IS WHY WE CAN'T HAVE NICE THINGS! IT WILL ALL JUST SMELL LIKE ROTTEN MILK!" On hands and knees, I sop up the mess, yelling, "I DO NOT EXIST TO CLEAN UP YOUR MESSES!"

Slightly terrified looks flash across my children's large, round, innocent eyes as they look sideways at one another, *Oh, boy. Here we go. Mom is losing it.* But on and on the rage flows from my chest until the milk is gone and our $179, totally replaceable blue-and-rust-colored rug is fine. It's clean. Then the guilt sets in, and I'm never a bit surprised when my period begins the following day. I hate that.

Rage is my least favorite part about womanhood and midlife. Also, most people forget to mention it, so we constantly feel like we're the only ones to occasionally lose our minds, use profanity with our boss, or basically terrorize our children over a cup of spilled milk. But we're not. I can assure you we're not the only ones to feel the flash of rage that is often hormonally related. More than 75% of women suffer from **premenstrual syndrome (PMS)** symptoms during the five days leading up to a menstrual period and have had similar monthly symptoms since their twenties (which means you've had roughly three hundred or more episodes of "losing it" due to PMS).[1] Up to 8% of women suffer from a more severe and debilitating form of PMS called **premenstrual dysphoric disorder (PMDD)**, which can often be described as rage.[2] Turns out we're not "losing it"; our bodies have only been temporarily taken over by hormones.

Digging Deeper into PMDD

Remember the hypothalamus and pituitary gland in the brain that work together on a feedback loop to control the release of hormones from the thyroid? The hypothalamus and pituitary gland also work together to stimulate the ovaries to make estrogen and progesterone and to develop a follicle in the ovary that will later release an egg during ovulation.

The first half of the menstrual cycle is called the **follicular phase**. During this time, **follicle-stimulating hormone (FSH)**, a hormone from the pituitary gland, begins telling the ovary to develop one main follicle, which contains an egg. And at the same time, the lining of the uterus, called the **endometrium**, thickens in response to rising levels of estrogen. Around day fourteen, when estrogen levels are high enough, ovulation occurs in response to a surge of a second hormone from the pituitary gland called **luteinizing hormone (LH)**.

The second half of the menstrual cycle is called the **luteal phase**. During this time, levels of estrogen drop sharply after ovulation then begin a slow and moderate rise. Progesterone levels from the now-empty follicle in the ovary progressively rise and peak, which helps to stabilize the endometrium and prepare a healthy lining within the uterus for a possibly fertilized egg to implant during pregnancy. Without fertilization and without the necessary signaling from an embryo to indicate pregnancy, levels of both progesterone and estrogen drop, and the endometrium is then shed during **menses** (the fancy word for a period) as the menstrual cycle begins all over again.[3]

The following graph provides a visual overview of the coordinating hormone levels during the menstrual cycle along with the associated changes in the endometrium:[4]

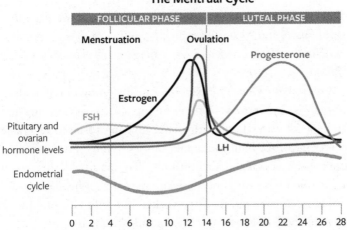

The most common symptoms of PMS include emotional and behavioral symptoms of depression, irritability, and increased anxiety along with physical complaints like breast pain, bloating, and headache. Symptoms recur monthly at the end of the luteal phase and resolve with the onset of menses.

Perhaps until now, you've had normal periods with mild PMS, but since turning forty, you're wondering what the heck is going on. Turns out, the menstrual cycle *changes* in our **later reproductive years**. The follicular phase shortens, and the time between cycles lessens by a few days. Menstrual bleeding may grow heavier (much heavier) and last longer (several days longer). And some women experience a worsening of PMS and PMDD symptoms with an increased risk for developing mood disorders during this time.[5]

It might look something like this:

A *day-to-day calendar of events for the midlife menstrual cycle and PMDD (along with a few simple recommendations for survival)*

Day 1: Your period begins—levels of estrogen and progesterone are low.

You might be thinking: *Oh, my period! I wondered when that would finally start! I should probably apologize to my family for my behavior these last few days. Where's the Tylenol? My head is killing me!*

Ways to help: Get some exercise. It really doesn't matter what, just get out and move your body. Fill up a sixty-four-oz. jug and drink lots of water. Eat healthy(ish) by having a fruit or vegetable at every meal, and limit your intake of sugar. Aim for seven to eight hours of sleep per night. Take an anti-inflammatory like ibuprofen (if you don't have any contraindications) for your headache. And apologize to your family or coworkers for your out-of-control behavior these last few days. Maybe call a friend to vent.

Insight for your spouse: At the onset of her period, your wife may feel terrible. It's likely she has a headache, and everything hurts. Sex is probably off limits, but you can help her symptoms by rubbing her neck and shoulders, then offering to pick up takeout for dinner.

Insight for your kids: Sweethearts, your mom has a killer headache. Try to keep it down, play nicely, and mostly stay out of her way.

Days 2–4: A ridiculously heavy menstrual period ensues.

You might be thinking: *This bleeding is NO JOKE. I can't go anywhere! How much more can I possibly lose? I am surely anemic. I better eat something with iron. Exercise sounds terrible; why do they always tell us to do that? My back hurts. My cramps hurt. I mostly just want to sit on the couch and eat bread or chocolate.*

Ways to help: See day 1. Also, please note that if you have a super-soaker bleeding event in which you are soaking through a pad or tampon in less than an hour and/or passing clots larger than a quarter, you need to call your doctor.

Insight for your spouse and kids: See day 1.

Day 5 or 6: Your period tricks you into thinking it is over.

Day 7: Light spotting continues for what feels like forever.

Days 8–10: You have a few precious days of totally normal.

You can remember things! You can complete tasks! You can read and learn new material! You can pick the kids up from school and somehow manage to field every single, "Hey mom! Guess what!" amid the bickering on the way home in the car.

Everyone: Simply enjoy this time.

Days 11–14: Ovulation occurs—estrogen levels have surged but begin to drop rapidly.

You might be thinking: *I feel amazing! I AM amazing! I am having such a good hair day. I look hot! I AM a little hot (and bothered). Where's my husband? Awwww . . . look at that baby. We should have another baby. We could totally have another baby. I want to do ALL the things! I should go back to work. Or maybe I should go back to school? I should sign up for a half-marathon. Or maybe I should sign up to be PTA president at the kids' school? I know, I should write a book. I am invincible! I am going to set this world on FIRE!*

Ways to help: Go do all the things and set the world on fire! You really are amazing!

Insight for your spouse: Walk up behind your wife this morning and kiss her neck then tell her she's beautiful. I almost guarantee she'll meet you in the shower or the closet or be waiting to pounce when you come to bed. *This* is the sex people talk about in middle age. (Please remember she can still get pregnant, so be sure the two of you have planned accordingly because right now her brain is clouded with precious baby thoughts.) Also, if you've been waiting to bring up an out-of-town trip or a puppy or that new electric car, this is the time to discuss it. She's confident she can handle *anything* right now.

Insight for your kids: My dears, your mom only has precious and loving thoughts for you, and you can do no wrong. If you've been wanting to ask for something, now is the time.

Days 15–22: You have a few precious days of totally normal— progesterone levels begin to climb and estrogen moderately increases.

You're not setting the world on fire necessarily, but you're getting things done. This part goes by in a blink.

Again, everyone: Enjoy this time and your wonderful, amazing, relatively stable wife and mom!

Days 23–28: PMS hits *hard*—Estrogen levels begin to decline, and progesterone reaches a peak then plummets, causing breast tenderness, bloating, weight gain, cravings, and a return of emotional lability.

You might be thinking: *What in the world is wrong with people? This place is a disaster! Why do we own all this STUFF? I'm the only one who does anything around here, and maybe I should just burn the whole house to the ground. Nothing can be salvaged. The kids are awful. My life is awful. And my husband doesn't notice anything I do. Plus, he can't possibly be attracted to me anymore. Look at this bloated tummy! None of my clothes fit. And look at this skin! Who has acne as a forty-four-year-old woman? Also, I'm starving. I am either going to run away from home or curl up into a ball and die!*

Ways to help: Survive. Do NOT burn the house to the ground. Try not to use profanity with your boss (or anyone else for that matter), and instead cover *everything* with grace. Maybe go out for a long, brisk walk. Let your legs pump away until you almost can't catch your breath (remember, this will help you complete the stress cycle). Healthy foods, water, and adequate sleep are *essential* during this time. Make a mental note to ask God one day why in the world He made hormones and periods this way.

Insight for your spouse: Tread lightly. Yes, this is probably PMS (or PMDD) talking, but you absolutely *cannot* mention that. Tell your wife she's beautiful and you love her and you know she's an amazing mom, and she might avoid crying in the closet. Also, remind her of that thing you just talked about this morning (and five minutes ago). Her hormones are all over the place, her brain is in a fog, and she can't remember a thing. If you are interested in sex, you better get to work on those dishes and plan on giving her a very long back rub. Also, don't forget to bring home takeout tomorrow.

Insight for your kids: I know, darlings, your mom doesn't seem like herself right now. Go play outside and absolutely stay out of her way. I promise she loves you to the moon. You can discuss it all with your therapist one day.

Return back to Day 1: Your period begins all over again!

Now, repeat this cycle ad nauseum until perimenopause begins to wreak further havoc (don't worry, we'll dive headfirst into perimenopause in chapter 7).

PMDD must be differentiated from psychiatric illness, a thyroid problem, the hormonal changes of the menopausal transition, or an underlying mood disorder like depression or dysthymia. Similar to PMS, PMDD symptoms occur in the three- to five-day window prior to menses and completely resolve once menses begins.

Symptoms of PMDD fit into two categories[6]

AFFECTIVE (AS IN MOOD OR FEELINGS) SYMPTOMS

- Mood swings, intense sadness, and vulnerability to rejection
- Anger, irritability, and outbursts

- Depressed mood, feelings of hopelessness, and self-critical thoughts
- Increased anxiety and feeling on edge

PHYSICAL SYMPTOMS

- Difficulty concentrating or "brain fog"
- Diminished interest in normal activities
- Change in appetite and increased cravings
- Fatigue
- Feeling "out of control"
- Breast tenderness, bloating, weight gain, muscle/joint pain

After a detailed history and evaluation of medications such as oral contraceptives that may contribute to the above symptoms plus laboratory work to rule out a thyroid disorder and check for anemia as a result of the increased bleeding with menses, the diagnosis of PMDD can be made after tracking symptoms over a two-month time frame and confirming that symptoms resolve completely during the follicular phase of the cycle. It is important to reliably track your symptoms, usually with a tool called the **Daily Record of Severity of Problems**.[7] If five or more symptoms are present during the week prior to menses and resolve when menses begins, then the diagnosis of PMDD is confirmed.

Focus on Healing

PMDD can be treated in a number of ways. If symptoms are mild, regular aerobic exercise combined with relaxation techniques and supplementation with chasteberry (vitex agnus-castus) may be beneficial. Unlike other supplements marketed for relieving PMS-like symptoms (such as primrose oil, vitamin B6, high-dose calcium, vitamin E, and magnesium), chasteberry has some good evidence through reliable studies that it reduces symptoms more than a placebo without any harmful side effects, though mild weight gain may occur.[8] Some women find relief from their symptoms with a combined (meaning it contains both estrogen and progesterone) oral birth control pill, though for others PMS and PMDD symptoms can worsen on the pill. All treatments will involve a little trial and error.

For more serious symptoms, selective serotonin reuptake inhibitors (SSRI) are highly effective for treating both PMS and PMDD. These include Lexapro, Celexa, Zoloft, Paxil, and Prozac. Some women find relief by taking an SSRI during only the luteal phase (or the second half of the cycle after ovulation occurs) of the cycle. Others require continuous treatment with an SSRI for complete symptom relief.[9] The most common side effect of SSRIs is related to decreased libido, delayed orgasm, or anorgasmia (the inability to achieve orgasm). These side effects are generally dose specific.

You can use the Daily Record of Severity of Symptoms chart in appendix 2 to track any symptoms associated with your menstrual cycle to be discussed with your healthcare provider. PMS, PMDD, and rage are common, but there are many options for help with these symptoms. Your provider is the best source of information for questions and concerns related to your symptoms and treatment of possible PMS or PMDD.

7

WHAT TO EXPECT IN PERIMENOPAUSE

A Guide to Hormones, Hot Flashes, and "The Change"

Being in my mid-forties means the things that used to work have mostly stopped working—my low-carb diet, our family's chore charts, my meal plan and weekly routines, my period tracker, and my bad habit of staying up way too late for just one more episode of *The Office*.

Suddenly I'm gaining weight, I'm not sleeping as soundly, I'm more forgetful sometimes, my children are growing and operating on their own schedules, I'm utterly exhausted, and I'm never sure who will be around for dinner. *Will we have all seven of us tonight or only three around the table? Did they tell me? Who knows? And how do I accommodate for that?* I mostly throw soups or pulled pork in the crockpot and assume everyone will just eat whenever they get home.

But when did these things change? When did I slip into this midlife mom-bod, unable to lose a few pounds in a week by running a couple miles and focusing on healthy eating? How long have I been this tired? When did it become hard to jog the three miles around the path by our house or piggy-back my youngest child around the yard? When did I start waking with a sore back in the morning? When, exactly, did my breasts begin their downward descent? And when did it become the norm to check in with my kids via text to see what they have going on for the day?

Do you work today?
Will you be home after school?
What time is practice? Do you need a ride?
Should I count on you for dinner?

I was once the vibrant and energetic CEO of our large family company, but lately all the inner workings of this well-oiled machine have been outsourced. People told me all along that motherhood is working myself out of a job, and this is what's *supposed* to happen. But where does that leave me when it's done? Am I taking early retirement? I'm not really sure, but I do know I am *so* tired.

My days are overflowing with laundry and schedules and emails and agendas and sports practices, and I spend a ridiculous amount of effort attempting to keep a gallon of milk in the house. It all feels mostly out of my control; like life is just . . . happening.

I asked my readers recently, *What is the hardest part about midlife?* And I received nearly a thousand answers that sounded like some version of this:

I went hiking with my daughter the other day and tore the medial meniscus in my knee. It wasn't even anything strenuous! I'm not sure what's happening. Until now, I've always been relatively fit. Is this really just my body now?

Being in my mid-forties with anxiety and a newly empty nest makes me feel so alone sometimes. Plus, women wear a lot of masks on social media like, "Life is great!" or "I'm super woman. I can do it ALL myself!" And it just adds to my loneliness.

I'm forty-five years old and parenting two teenage girls. Life is so busy right now! My days are filled with work, and evenings and weekends are spent in a mad dash running around to the girls' sports. I am struggling with not feeling like myself from heavy periods that are coming closer together, breakouts (I thought I was done with those years ago), insomnia, hot flashes, low libido, and weight gain. Plus, I recently got shingles. Am I old enough to get shingles? On top of that my parents seem to be rapidly aging, and I'm trying to help them as much as I can. This part of life is stressful to say the least! The hardest part about midlife is not just *one* thing . . . it's ALL of it.

At almost fifty-two, this perimenopause business is no joke! I'm experiencing sheer exhaustion. Plus, as a Black woman, I often feel like my symptoms are dismissed by medical providers because of the color of my skin, and I'm frustrated. Women are not meant to simply suck it up and suffer through this!

Just the sight of people (like my husband and kids) in my clean kitchen cooking breakfast is making me act really mean, and I suspect it's not them. It's me. I feel so angry most of the time!

My forties are already nothing like I expected. It feels like my whole system is on fire! I'm hoping to turn it around and learn how to live with it in a realistic way. Really, I just want to find some comfort and peace.

Most of us enter midlife and the hormonal chaos of perimenopause feeling duped because until now we've been promised a set of rules with predictable outcomes. We've inadvertently absorbed the marketing and those empty promises of the "beauty and wellness" industry, and unbeknownst to most of us, we've been living assuredly within a When/Then theology all our lives, believing:

When the kids get older . . .
When I lose ten pounds . . .

When we move into a bigger or better house . . .

When I start my new job or finish school or cut down to part time or finally get to stay home with the kids . . .

When I fit into those old jeans . . .

When I find the right diet or the right exercise program or the perfect "natural" supplement for these hot flashes . . .

When I get this house decluttered or organized or updated or decorated . . .

When all the kids are in school or when school gets out or when summer is over . . .

When I can do something about this stomach flab or maybe get more muscle definition . . .

When I finish this or that or get through my never-ending to-do list . . .

Then I'll have more time.

Then we will finally have a chance to travel.

Then I'll be able to relax a little and slow down.

Then life will be easier.

Then I'll be beautiful. And my *life* will be beautiful.

Then I'll finally feel caught up.

Then I'll be successful.

Then I might actually be *happy*.

Then I can breeeeeaaaathe.

But despite what we've been told, life doesn't have a plateau. There just isn't a place where one day we'll arrive and it's all coasting after that. Relaxing. From what I understand, we don't ever *get there*. Things continually . . . change.

Our relationships change. Our job descriptions change. Our roles as a parent and spouse and daughter and sister and friend and coworker and neighbor change. Our children grow and move away and begin their own adult lives with spouses and jobs and children and roles of their own. Our parents fall ill or die. Our spouses develop chronic illness. Our energy diminishes. Our bodies change and begin to fail. Everything we once knew eventually changes. We simply . . . change. And it doesn't mean we're doing anything wrong; it means we're living a life. All the things we've worked for, hoped for, strived for over the years will fade. And we will have to let go again and again and again. Whatever it is we're holding in a death grip right now will change. Life itself is *change*.

And it makes me wonder why we aren't talking more about it. Why aren't we sharing the truth about the inevitable changes we *all* face in midlife? More specifically, why aren't we talking about "The Change"?

Digging Deeper into Perimenopause

I teach maturation class every year to fifth-grade students at an elementary school in our community. On some random Tuesday every April, a group of round-faced, nervous-looking students gather hesitantly in a classroom along with the parents (those parents who can manage to take the morning off from work), and together we watch a cheesy, after-school-special kind of film about girls and boys their age going through puberty. There are little vignettes showing friends at school or the tragic story of starting a period at a sleepover or examples of kids navigating the puberty transition with a single parent of the opposite sex. And in between the stories, animated cartoon diagrams demonstrate the way hormones are released from the ovaries or testes after a signal is given from the brain, then circulate throughout the body and produce the typical changes of puberty like development of hair in the armpits and pubic areas, breast buds and other secondary sex characteristics, boys' erections, and a girl's first menstrual period.

After the video, we talk about the *range of normal* and what the kids can expect as they go through their own change toward an adult body. The students usually glance around red-faced and embarrassed and roll their eyes at their friends and giggle in all the right places. But mostly, year after year they are genuinely engaged. They really *do* want to know what to expect from puberty.

I pass out little strips of paper for them to write down anonymous questions, then I answer the questions aloud for the group. I add details from my own list to make sure we cover everything they need to know, and I include tips for parents that will spur further conversations at home. We briefly discuss sex, pregnancy, sexually transmitted disease prevention, and the topic of consent. And after our two-hour session, I pass out a bag of goodies with handouts, mini sticks of deodorant, and sample menstrual products for the girls.

Throughout my presentation, the principal stands quietly at the back of the room next to the teachers who are in attendance, along with the school secretary. All the parents seated around the room smile and nod knowingly throughout our discussion. Afterward, they hug their children goodbye and head back to work. And the whole event is like a little rite of passage. An initiation into the inevitable hormonal chaos of puberty. In this coming-of-age affair about the normal transition from childhood into the teen years and on into adulthood, a supportive community of people who love these budding young tweens and who have been in their relatively awkward, pre-adolescent shoes gather around to show our love and share what we know through experience about this next stage of life.

Though the students tend to dread this day—and of course giggle and laugh and roll their eyes and groan—they leave with the reassuring knowledge of what is to come. They feel empowered, and they are relieved to know that puberty is common, expected, and manageable. Plus, they understand there is a group of knowledgeable, loving adults who care and want to support them all the way through.

I like to think of menopause as puberty except in reverse.

Menopause, too, is a universal experience for all women with ovaries who live long enough to reach the menopausal years. Unfortunately, many women are not well informed about the physical changes or symptoms that come with fluctuations in hormones, the ongoing medical effects caused by decreased levels of estrogen and other hormones in their bodies, and the treatment options available to them. There isn't a rite of passage or initiation into the inevitable hormonal chaos of the menopausal transition. No one is telling us that menopause is common, expected, and manageable. And instead, many women's symptoms and health concerns related to menopause are dismissed and ignored, or worse, pathologized and exploited in the name of money by the "wellness" industry.

The truth is most women will spend up to *one half of their lives* in the perimenopausal transition and postmenopausal years. So, I think it's time we talk openly and honestly about it, don't you?

The hormonal changes of perimenopause can trigger a variety of symptoms[1]

- Abnormal menstrual bleeding in the form of heavy or irregular periods, skipped periods, or bleeding between periods
- Hot flashes and night sweats, which may include palpitations or an irregular heartbeat
- Weight gain
- Changes in sleep (especially frequent nighttime waking)
- Cognitive changes (i.e., the dreaded brain fog)
- Hair loss and changes in hair texture
- Adult acne
- Thinning of vaginal mucosa and dryness causing pain with sex
- Decreased libido and/or a decreased ability to achieve orgasm

- Joint pain and stiffness
- Itching or ringing in the ears

On top of that, the hormonal changes of menopause can also be associated with a variety of other medical illnesses

- Cardiovascular disease
- Osteoporosis
- Depression
- Type 2 diabetes
- Metabolic syndrome
- Dementia
- Urinary tract infections

When the symptoms of perimenopause appear on top of any *other* underlying medical conditions like hypothyroidism, depression, or autoimmune disease, plus any normal changes associated with aging and a myriad of other environmental and social factors concurrently changing in midlife, then it can *all* feel like . . . well . . . chaos. Right?

Wouldn't it be nice if there was a "menopause class" to answer all your questions? And even better, wouldn't it be great to join in a gathering of supportive and loving women who might smile and nod knowingly as they pass along their wisdom because they've *all* been in your shoes? If we were together in a classroom today, what questions would you write down on your little scrap of paper? Let me answer some of the most common questions women have about menopause.

What do you mean by the term perimenopause? *Isn't menopause a one-time event?*

Menopause is marked by a **final menstrual period (FMP)**, the last period you will ever have. Unfortunately, we can't know which period is the official last one until twelve months *after* that final period. When a woman has gone twelve months without any menstrual bleeding, menopause can be confirmed in *retrospect*. The **menopausal transition**, then, is the four to ten years of hormonal fluctuations and bodily changes leading up to the FMP. You probably know that the prefix *peri* means around. **Perimenopause**, then, includes both the menopausal transition and the first year after menopause is confirmed, or "the time around" menopause.

Early in the menopausal transition, cycles may begin lengthening by a week or more with occasional skipped periods. Later into the menopausal transition, skipped periods become more common. When two periods in a row are missed, the FMP is likely to occur within the next four years.[2] The timing of the menopausal transition and the FMP is highly variable from woman to woman, making unpredictability the very most predictable part of menopause.

Which hormones are involved in the menopausal transition?

Hormones are known as the "chemical messengers" of the body, relaying messages from place to place and controlling bodily functions. Several hormones are involved in the changes of perimenopause, and fluctuations in these hormones can trigger the variety of symptoms mentioned above. Three of the hormones that we already discussed in chapter 6 are the *key contributors* in the menopausal transition:

1. **Estradiol** is mostly produced by the ovary in the developing follicle that releases an egg at ovulation. A small amount of estradiol is also produced in fat, bone, muscle, liver, and brain tissue. Levels of estradiol vary throughout the normal menstrual cycle and can range from 30 pg/ml in the early follicular phase up to 300 pg/ml at ovulation. During the menopausal transition, estradiol released

from the ovary drops significantly to <25 pg/ml after menopause.

2. **Progesterone** is produced by the ovary in the empty follicle after ovulation occurs, and the levels of progesterone decline throughout the menopausal transition.

3. **Follicle Stimulating Hormone (FSH)** from the pituitary gland regulates ovulation and subsequently the levels of estradiol and progesterone. FSH levels begin to rise during the menopausal transition, and after menopause the level of FSH will be >30 IU/ml.[3]

When will I begin menopause? How will I know? Is there a blood test to see where I'm at?

The average age of menopause is 51 years, and the biggest contributor to the timing of *your* menopause is genetics. Black women will generally have a longer menopausal transition than white women with a higher incidence of vasomotor symptoms, which we'll talk about in more detail later. Most women will follow a similar menstrual path as their mother and sisters, though other factors play a part. A variety of environmental, social, and economic factors such as a personal history of smoking, a lower socioeconomic status, a history of other chronic medical illnesses, and poorer overall health can significantly impact the timing of menopause.

Unfortunately, there isn't a blood test to "see where you're at." Levels of estradiol, progesterone, and FSH vary *significantly* both from day to day within a cycle *and* from cycle to cycle. A random sample of blood work revealing a low estradiol and high FSH could be menopause, or it could be a result of one missed period. Furthermore, studies show that hormone levels do not correlate with a woman's symptoms. So, for all these reasons, "**hormone levels should not be used to predict the timing of the final menstrual period, diagnose menopause, or to guide therapy for women** over the age of forty."[4] I realize that repeated hormone testing may provide the illusion that a provider is listening and individualizing therapy; however, such tests simply add unnecessary expense through repeated office visits, repeated blood work, and repeated adjustments to medication based on results that we already know *will* fluctuate.

Instead, both the diagnosis and treatment of perimenopause should be based on *symptoms*. A woman in her forties or early fifties with irregular periods and symptoms such as hot flashes, weight changes, brain fog, and the others mentioned above is clearly in her menopausal transition and should be treated with medication based on her preferences without requiring a hormone level for diagnosis or following a particular blood level for treatment.

What is happening during a hot flash?

The symptoms of hot flashes and night sweats can be lumped together into something called **vasomotor symptoms (VMS)**, which affect 80% of women during perimenopause and beyond. Hot flashes typically feel like a sudden and intense feeling of heat over the head, neck, chest, and arms along with sweating and redness of the face and chest. VMS may also cause uncontrollable anxiety, nausea, and even an irregular heartbeat.[5]

Hot flashes are caused by something called **thermoregulatory dysfunction** in the hypothalamus of the brain due to withdrawal of estrogen. To eliminate all this extra heat, the blood vessels in the skin dilate (or open up) to cause flushing, and the sweat glands begin to perspire. Most hot flashes last around four minutes, and generally chills and shivering immediately follow to bring the body temperature back to normal. Usually, hot flashes are relatively unpredictable, but they can sometimes be brought on by heat, activity, spicy foods, caffeine, alcohol, and stressful situations. Regardless of the trigger, these episodes can occur up to thirty times a day, and on average, episodes of hot flashes can last for up to seven years of the menopausal transition. Yikes!

Hot flashes that occur at night can cause intense sweating with soaked sheets, frequent nighttime waking, and anxiety—all just another contributor to our difficulty with sleep during midlife.

There are other possible causes of sweating and hot flashes, so conditions like carcinoid syndrome, hyperthyroidism, infection, anxiety, cancer, and medication side effects must be ruled out before any treatment for menopausal hot flashes can begin.

Mild symptoms from hot flashes can be treated by lowering the room temperature, dressing in layers, using fans, avoiding alcohol and spicy foods, and decreasing stress and anxiety. More severe symptoms that haven't improved with nonmedication options can be relieved with prescription medications like menopausal hormone therapy, antidepressants, antiepileptic drugs like Gabapentin, or a blood pressure medication called Clonidine. Fezolinetant (Veozah) is a new medication released in 2023 specifically designed to reduce flushing and sweating spells.

Many "natural" supplements like black cohosh, cannabis, phytoestrogens, vitamin E, and evening primrose oil have been poorly studied, so they lack evidence-based support and may contain variable dosing or additional contaminants. These supplements are generally not recommended.[6] More on supplements to come.

What's up with all this bleeding?

Menstrual irregularity is the hallmark sign of the menopausal transition. Bleeding is labeled abnormal when it becomes heavy (which is called **menorrhagia**) or does not follow a regular pattern, resulting in longer periods, irregular cycles, and bleeding between cycles (which is called **metrorrhagia**). The amount of blood shed during a menstrual period typically increases during the menopausal transition, and it can suddenly be common to leak through menstrual products, pass clots, or bleed for longer than seven days.[7]

In general, abnormal bleeding results from the hormonal chaos of the menopausal transition; however, there are other causes of abnormal bleeding such as **uterine fibroids** (termed **leiomyomas**) or **adenomyosis** (when the endometrium, or lining of the uterus, begins to invade the muscular wall of the uterus).

Evaluation of bleeding during the menopausal transition includes a pelvic exam, blood work to rule out an unexpected pregnancy and evaluate the function of both the thyroid and the pituitary gland with various hormone levels, an ultrasound to look at the thickness of the uterine lining and rule out fibroids or adenomyosis, and a possible tissue sampling of the endometrium of the uterus called an **endometrial biopsy**.

If abnormal bleeding is a result of hormonal changes related to the menopausal transition, there are many available interventions for treatment:[8]

1. Tranexamic acid works on clotting to decrease the amount of bleeding when taken for the first five days of menstrual bleeding.
2. Estrogen-containing products can regulate the menstrual cycle, decrease bleeding, and help with cramping and hot flashes. We'll talk more about estrogen and other hormones below.
3. The Levonorgestrel intrauterine device (IUD) reduces bleeding and may halt periods altogether.
4. Over-the-counter (OTC) nonsteroidal anti-inflammatory medications (NSAIDS) like ibuprofen can help both with bleeding and cramping.
5. Hysterectomy removes the uterus completely and is the definitive procedure for abnormal bleeding.

All bleeding that occurs *after* the final menstrual period (remember menopause means twelve months with no bleeding, a diagnosis made in retrospect) is referred to as **postmenopausal bleeding** and is considered *abnormal*. Postmenopausal bleeding *must* be evaluated with blood work, an ultrasound, and an endometrial biopsy by your healthcare provider.[9]

Why is it so dang hard to lose weight?

Weight gain is common during midlife and perimenopause, and oftentimes losing weight by the methods that used to work seems much harder than it was previously. Loss of muscle mass begins in our mid-thirties and forties, and since muscles are responsible for burning calories and energy consumption, this change in overall muscle mass may contribute to the "slowing of metabolism" many women believe comes with middle age. Furthermore, genetics, stress, poor sleep, depression, changes in diet and activity level, and medications taken for chronic illnesses like antidepressants, insulin, oral steroids, and beta-blockers can all contribute to weight gain.

Most women will see an increase in abdominal and **visceral fat** (the fat within the abdomen surrounding the internal organs). This increase in visceral fat increases the risk of cardiovascular disease in midlife and is one component for the diagnosis of **metabolic syndrome.**[10] When three out of five of the following markers are present, a diagnosis of metabolic syndrome can be made, which increases the risk for heart disease, stroke, and type 2 diabetes:

- A waist circumference >88 cm
- A high triglyceride level (which is a component of the total cholesterol)
- A low HDL (which is the body's *good* cholesterol)
- A diagnosis of high blood pressure (measuring >140/90 on two occasions)
- A consistently high blood sugar (>100 when measured fasting)

We can preserve our muscle mass and reduce the risk for metabolic syndrome through both regular exercise that includes weightlifting *and* healthy diet choices, which we'll discuss further in chapter 12 when we talk about preventative health.

Am I at risk for depression during menopause?

Depression is experienced as sadness that won't go away, decreased interest or pleasure in activities that were previously enjoyed, a general feeling of hopelessness, and lasting low energy levels. Women tend to have higher rates of depression compared to men, and the hormonal changes of perimenopause can trigger depression to emerge, especially in women who are already at risk. We will talk more about the symptoms, screening and diagnosis, and various treatments for depression and other common mood disorders in chapter 9.[11]

I can't remember a single thing. Is this just my brain now?

"Brain fog" is real. In the Study of Women's Health Across the Nation (SWAN) study, two-thirds of women reported cognitive difficulties during perimenopause. They described memory concerns, forgetfulness, trouble with word finding, and an inability to stay focused and complete a task. The study showed an overall impact on the participants' ability to take in and retain new information. But after following study participants over several years, the SWAN study further revealed that changes in brain functioning due to the hormonal changes of perimenopause were *temporary* and disappeared once women became postmenopausal.[12]

Hormones are not the only factor affecting our brains. Mood disorders like depression or anxiety, sleep issues like insomnia or sleep apnea, and other chronic illnesses can also contribute to problems with "brain fog." And hey, remember our old friend *stress*? Midlife is a time for huge shifts in motherhood roles, increased caregiver functions, changes in career paths, marital issues, financial burdens, and more. Women in midlife experience incredible amounts of stress. It's no wonder we can't find our car keys!

Hormonal therapy may improve the symptoms of "brain fog"; however, other contributing factors like thyroid disease, type 2 diabetes, sleep apnea, and mood disorders must first be ruled out. Focusing on healthy eating and regular exercise, plus finding strategies for relieving or coping with midlife stress will also help. It may help to remember that the "brain fog" of perimenopause is temporary, but you might consider a referral from your primary provider for formal neuropsychiatric testing if your cognitive function seems to worsen drastically.

Is there anything I can DO about the symptoms of perimenopause?

Non-estrogen therapies are available to treat the individual symptoms of perimenopause. Hot flashes may improve with non-medical treatments like environmental changes (dressing in layers, lowering the temperature, avoiding triggers, etc.) and with prescription medications like SSRIs, antiepileptics, and/or Clonidine or Veozah as mentioned earlier. Vaginal dryness or other vaginal symptoms may be treated with vaginal lubricants and moisturizers, which are available over the counter. In addition, prescription vaginal estrogen cream can be used topically with a much lower side-effect profile than oral estrogen and without the accompanying use of progesterone.

Other perimenopausal symptoms like anxiety, brain fog, and changes in sleep/libido can be improved with a variety of treatment options like exercise, healthy diet, antidepressants, stress reduction, proper sleep hygiene, and/or a visit with a sex therapist. We will discuss each of these in depth throughout this book.

And finally, if non-estrogen therapies do not prove beneficial, many women find relief from their perimenopausal symptoms through treatment with estrogen (which may require accompanying progesterone) in what is referred to as **menopausal hormone therapy (MHT)**.[13]

Estrogen is a safe, effective, and often underutilized treatment for relief of menopausal symptoms and comes in two forms:

1. **Transdermal estrogen** is absorbed through the skin via a patch, gel, spray, or vaginal ring providing a consistent low level of estrogen to the bloodstream with a lower risk profile. Several doses are available so therapy can be customized to each woman's needs.

2. **Oral estrogen** is typically given in the form of estradiol at variable doses.

Rather than achieve an estrogen level similar to pre-menopause, the lowest dose of estrogen necessary to provide relief of perimenopausal *symptoms* is the treatment goal.

Progestin (a progesterone-like hormone) must be given together with estrogen if a uterus is present because estrogen given alone (termed **unopposed estrogen**) is a risk factor for developing endometrial cancer. To protect the uterus, progestin must be given for at least twelve days per cycle. It can be taken orally or given in the form of an IUD. For some women in their forties with symptoms during the menopausal transition, a low-dose oral birth control pill containing both estrogen and progesterone is effective and can also protect against pregnancy.

In general, MHT is a safe treatment option for healthy, symptomatic women who are younger than age 60 and within ten years of menopause. MHT is associated with a small increased risk of certain estrogen-receptor-positive breast cancers, stroke, blood clots, and gallbladder disease. Women who are already at higher risk for these conditions need to weigh the risks and benefits of MHT carefully.

Use of testosterone for perimenopausal women is considered "off-label" for treatment of anything other than decreased libido; however, for certain symptoms and certain individuals, testosterone may be beneficial. You can talk with your personal healthcare provider for more information. I believe this is an area where we'll see developing treatments coming soon.

Contraindications to hormone therapy (meaning in general it should either NOT be used or used with caution after an informed discussion with your provider) may include[14]

- Current or past history of certain types of breast cancer
- Current or past history of endometrial cancer
- Known coronary heart disease
- Active liver disease
- History of a blood clot, stroke, or transient ischemic attack
- Any woman at high risk for these complications

My friend takes a "menopause" supplement recommended by her homeopathic provider. Should I be taking that? Isn't there something more "natural" I can use like those bioidenticals I keep hearing about?

More than 75% of women will turn to alternative therapies for treatment of menopausal symptoms. Though individual studies may show some benefit to several alternative therapies, the sample sizes in these studies are frequently small, and the duration of treatment is relatively short. Furthermore, the placebo given in such studies shows a benefit in up to 50% of study subjects, which proves that simple *belief* in a treatment may be enough to produce the desired effect. Accompanying studies on the safety and efficacy of many of these alternative therapies, however, have not been well established, and often treatment (with bioidentical hormones especially) is misunderstood. I will discuss a few of the most-used "alternative" therapies for perimenopausal symptoms in more detail here:[15]

1. **Phytoestrogens** are compounds found in plants that are often referred to as "plant-based hormones"; however, it is

important to note that they aren't actually hormones. Phy-toestrogens can mimic estrogen or interfere with estrogen by acting on the estrogen receptor, but our human bodies cannot convert plant compounds into hormones. Using phytoestrogens for treatment of perimenopausal symptoms has not been shown to cause harm; however, in reputable studies, treatment with phytoestrogens does not exhibit a proven or significant impact on the symptoms of perimenopause like hot flashes, vaginal dryness, or sleep quality.

2. **Bioidentical hormones** create a lot of confusion and refer to the *structure* of the hormones used for MHT. **Bioidentical hormones** have the same chemical and molecular structure as hormones produced by the human body, while **non-bioidentical hormones** are structurally dissimilar to the hormones produced by the human body but equally effective. Due to concerns about safety over the years (and very good marketing toward bioidenticals), bioidentical hormones (which are often incorrectly called "natural" hormones) have become increasingly popular.

Many women believe that bioidentical hormones must be prescribed by a holistic or alternative-type provider and that all prescription hormones from a conventional physician are synthetic and non-bioidentical, but this isn't true. A prescription from your primary medical provider can be either non-bioidentical or bioidentical, depending on the product prescribed.

Often the confusion comes from misunderstanding the difference between **compounded hormone therapy** and non-compounded FDA-approved prescription hormones. *All* bioidentical hormones (both the compounded and non-compounded FDA-approved varieties) are derived from a steroid in soy and yams, and *both* need to be commercially processed prior to use. Compounding pharmacies take processed bioidentical hormones derived from soy and yams and prepare, mix, assemble, and package the hormones into very patient-specific gels, creams, or other formulations. The non-compounded FDA-approved bioidentical hormones (which are *also* derived from soy and yams and processed *in the very same way*) are instead routed to pharmaceutical companies to be packaged into standard-dose formulations of pills, patches, gels, creams, sprays, or rings.[16]

Having FDA approval means a product has undergone extensive third-party testing and standardization regarding safety, efficacy, purity, potency, and consistency from batch to batch. Furthermore, ongoing post-marketing analysis done by the FDA continuously evaluates for adverse events. While custom compounded bioidentical hormones may undergo regulation by state boards of pharmacy, they *are not* subject to the same federal laws and *do not* have the ongoing systematic post-marketing analysis.

Compounded products purposefully contain different hormone combinations and delivery systems tailored for each patient; however, this highly specific individualization can lead to variation in absorption and inconsistencies from batch to batch in prescriptions refilled by that individual patient each month. Furthermore, because of this specialization, compounded products may not be covered by insurance and can be very pricey. For these reasons, conventional medicine does not routinely recommend compounded hormone products.

In short, you can get bioidentical FDA-approved hormones through a prescription from your conventional primary care provider. And as a bonus, these prescriptions are generally affordable, too!

3. **Herbal supplements** such as oxaloacetate with vitamin C for premenstrual symptoms, black cohosh for hot flashes, St. John's Wort for mood, chasteberry for menstrual

cramps and bloating, and literally thousands of other supplements are available over the counter with potential benefits for symptom relief based on thousands of studies of varying scale. However, the major issue with herbals and supplements is that they are widely *unregulated* since the Dietary Supplement Health and Education Act (DSHEA) passed in the United States, removing multiple safeguards for consumers.[17]

Those who push "natural" supplements will claim that "natural" is always superior treatment over "Big Pharma." This **appeal to nature** seems logical—if it's "natural" it must be good, and anything synthetic is bad. But this simply isn't true. We can point to thousands of examples. Sunlight is natural and helps provide vitamin D in the skin, but it can also cause all kinds of skin damage and lead to melanoma. Mushrooms grow naturally in the forest, yet some varieties are extremely poisonous to eat. What about earthquakes? Or tornadoes? They're natural . . . but can we call them good? On the other hand, vaccines are produced in mass quantities in a factory and responsible for reducing or even eliminating deadly diseases. And I personally watched and held a heart from a man's chest as replacement blood vessels were stitched in place while his blood and oxygen were exchanged using a cardiopulmonary bypass machine. Is there anything more *un*natural? And yet, how utterly amazing! Whether something is synthetic or natural is completely irrelevant. What matters is whether that particular product has been tested and proven safe for use in *humans*.

I am not anti-natural or anti-all-supplements; however, I *do* encourage information, critical thinking, understanding, and caution. We'll talk more about supplements (including the ones I recommend to my patients) and the three important questions to answer before beginning any medical intervention, including "natural" supplements, in chapter 11.

Focus on Healing

Listen, not every problem in midlife is due to perimenopause or hormones, because, remember? Midlife is not just *one* thing, it's *all* of it. And no one treatment is likely to "fix" the myriad complaints that come along with the mess.

We may never reach a plateau where life is free and easy in the way we always imagined it would be, but we *can* find health, healing, and wellness in the inevitable and endless change that flows our way. This next stage of life is the time to make decisions and develop best practices for your own specific circumstances based on the whole picture of your unique life. You can begin by slipping on that Control Filter and taking care of your ever-changing and evolving body the best way you know how.

Let's review where you can start

- Make mostly healthy food choices with a focus on at least one fruit or vegetable at every meal, lean protein, healthy fats, and whole grains. Consider the advice of a registered dietitian if you need additional help.
- Get regular aerobic exercise and include both flexibility/balance training and resistance training to help maintain your muscle mass and mobility.
- Complete the stress cycle through daily exercise, deep breathing, regular social interaction, and emotional or creative expression.
- Avoid smoking and limit alcohol use.
- Find support from your team—your family, friends, doctor, therapist or specialized support group, and more. We'll talk more about that in chapter 15.

- Work closely with your doctor and take individualized, FDA-approved medications for your specific perimeno-pausal symptoms when you need them.
- Prioritize sleep, aiming for seven to eight hours per night.

And remember, there is no one "right way."

My dear friend, *you are allowed to change*. You are allowed to change your mind. You are allowed to change in your appearance. You are allowed to change who you are. You are allowed to learn and grow and become a little more *you*—read new things, meet new people, experience new experiences. You are allowed to let go of cultural "beauty and wellness" expectations. You are allowed to look back at what you once felt or believed to be true and begin to believe something totally brand new. Midlife is full of change, and your medical provider can help you through it.

Now is the time, and you *can* do it. You are allowed to heal.

8

LOVING THE BODY
YOU *ACTUALLY* HAVE

I took a herd of kids swimming one day last summer—four of my own children along with two extra friends. When we entered the pool area, the kids sprinted away, laughing and splashing and cannonballing off the side and hollering, "Momma, watch! Look at me! Momma? Are you watching? Mooooom!"

I found a place in the shade for our bags and towels and sandals, looking up occasionally to smile and shout back, "Wow! That was a big splash! Great job!" And without really meaning to, I also noticed the other swimsuit-clad bodies of various ages and sizes pass by—young and full, chubby and limping, lean and muscled, droopy and shriveled with age, loose-skinned, taut-skinned, dark-skinned, fair-skinned, covered in hair or age spots, spilling over with rolls around the middle. As each uniquely human body walked by our little perch in the shade, I found myself thinking, *I wonder if that person has any idea how incredibly beautiful they are? How beloved, treasured, and adored? How perfectly loved in the eyes of God?* Then I peeled off my swimsuit cover-up and waddled to the pool with my doughy waistline and dimply thighs.

It was the first summer in a very long time that I had chosen a bikini for my summer suit (a bikini is more comfortable after all—easier bathroom access, less tugging and pulling). And it was the first year in my entire life that I wasn't slinking around the pool area in my new swimsuit hoping to reach the cover of my towel or searching for a dark corner of shade or walking swiftly with a small child in front of my body as a human shield, thinking, *Don't look at me. I'm repulsive!* It wasn't because I'd finally found the right diet plan to get to my optimal weight or finally started on an exercise program that produced a toned body with washboard abs. It's just that I am finally tired of mistreating myself. Tired of hating the packaging I come in. Tired of ridiculing this one precious, beautiful body in which I'm living out the days of my one precious, beautiful life—this body I *actually* have.

I stationed myself under the slide to catch little children flinging into the water with a splash when a woman about my age approached me from the side. "Excuse me. Maybe this is weird. . . ." She hesitated. "But I just wanted to say you are really beautiful."

I must've stared back at her with the expression of a blobfish—confused and a bit gelatinous. Then I glanced around at all the other women at the pool and blinked a few times before stammering, "What? Oh, umm. Thank you!"

"Yeah. I saw you walk in. Then I noticed you laughing with your kids, and I just had to come tell you. You're a *really* beautiful person."

I wasn't sure how to respond. My first instinct was to provide her with a list of evidence to the contrary—my large and saggy chest, my pudgy waistline, the wrinkles surrounding my eyes, the dull, peeling dry skin around my nose, the flesh rubbing together between my dimply thighs, my adult acne. I wanted to correct her or at least point her in the direction of a slimmer woman in the crowd, but instead (because I am just so tired of mistreating myself) I smiled and replied, "Wow. That's the nicest thing anyone has said to me in a long time. Thank you. I really appreciate you saying that!"

"Of course!" she flashed me a warm smile and swam off to the deep end to watch her own kids cannonballing off the side. I beamed. I am finally learning that if I cannot be okay—beautiful even—in this current body at this current weight with this imperfect skin and these dimply thighs, I won't be okay twenty pounds lighter. I just . . . won't.

✳ ✳ ✳ ✳

I told my sister on the phone the other day that I've been calling myself a well-being advocate because I believe that becoming well and finding healing and wholeness within the specific parameters each of us has been given is possibly the most important thing we can do in our lifetime. But I went on to say that if I'm really going to write about it and talk about it and even preach it a little, then I simply cannot continue to mistreat myself. I cannot continue to starve myself of entire food groups and belittle myself when I see my body reflected in the mirror. I cannot outwardly talk about love and bodily acceptance, then turn inward and hate myself in the same breath. I cannot be a hypocrite. And I am happy to report that I'm getting it right about 32% of the time (like that day at the pool). Today my **body image**, or the feelings I have about my body, is far from perfect, but it's a vast improvement from where I once was. In my mid-forties, I am better at simply *loving* my form.

The last time I can remember feeling truly accomplished about my body's appearance (because I had whittled it down to the cultural ideal) was seven years ago, when I had just weaned my youngest child from breastfeeding and was basically following a carb-free, no sugar, hyper-restrictive diet. Again. Back then, the familiar, ugly voice in my mind hissed at me regularly. *Ugh. You are so gross. Don't eat that. Why would you eat that? If you eat that you're going to be even fatter, you know. And you are already so disgusting. Put it down. You shouldn't eat one more thing for the rest of the day. You don't deserve to eat. Period.*

Then during a bout of viral gastroenteritis passed along from one of the kids, I found myself on the bathroom scale following hours of throwing up overnight. When the digital results flashed across the screen, I broke into a triumphant smile. It was an absolutely delightful number! And though I was exhausted and weak from dehydration, I crept into the closet and pulled an old pair of jeans that pre-dated my children from the bottom drawer. They were totally out of style with a hole along the inner seam, so I never wore them out and about, but I kept them tucked safely away for fifteen years and pulled them out occasionally to use as a barometer for my weight.

I was ecstatic to find that my old, pre-pregnancy jeans slipped easily over my thighs and hips, then buttoned at the waist with *extra* room. This was my pre-pregnancy weight! This was my exhausted, dehydrated, slightly starved, hyper-restricted pre-pregnancy body! I spun weakly in the mirror and cocked my hip into a sexy, disheveled-looking pose as I looped one finger through a beltloop. Those old jeans felt *so* good against my thin, bedraggled body. I popped some Tylenol to take the edge off my fever, managed a few sips of cool water, and dragged myself back to bed thinking, *I look amaaaaa-zing.* Then, feeling very pleased with myself, I attempted to sleep off the sickness.

I was thirty-seven years old, and I was still so lost.

The elation I felt that day was the same kind of elation I felt when I weighed myself in college after a particularly restrictive week without sugar or carbs or, basically, food (along with perhaps the occasional episode of purging in the bathroom of my sorority). And though I had gone on to become a mother of five children and worked as a family practice doctor who counseled people on healthy lifestyle practices—mindful food choices, exercise, rest, and hydration—I still *longed* to be thin. I longed to be one of those women who can eat whatever they want (which it turns out may just be a spinach salad with a dry chicken breast and a handful of almonds) and never have to experience the dreaded thigh rub or rolls of extra flesh flopping over the tops of their jeans. I desperately wanted *the fix* for what felt like my biggest flaw. My body.

Like all of us, I grew up in an appearance-focused world, bombarded with images portraying the cultural ideal of what it means to be a "beautiful" woman—rail-thin, toned, large and perkychested, curvy in all the right places without an inch of extra flesh, clear-skinned with soft and luscious long hair and rippling abs and provocative thighs. The world equates fitness with thinness, leading us to believe that healthy bodies *must* be thin. The thinner the better! So we engage in exercise and obsessive eating habits that prioritize the appearance of our bodies above all else.

We were taught nothing about health from the inside out, nothing about intuitive eating or trusting ourselves to think critically about how to care for our bodies with reasonable exercise and a variety of foods in moderation without guilt or shame. And instead, we were repeatedly blasted with comments our parents or neighbors or teachers or friends made about their bodies (or even our own bodies) alongside marketing ads featuring "ideal"-bodied, eternally young women with firm thighs and smooth foreheads—those ads peddling retinols and ceramides and replacement shakes and cool-sculpting all in the name of "beauty and wellness."

For many of us, it became terribly distressing that our own bodies were such an ordinary disaster. I know *I* never was all that thin or toned or clear skinned. I've never had rippling abs or provocative thighs. And though eventually I did become large chested, my breasts have always been slightly mismatched in size and drooping in all the wrong places (and mostly responsible for neck pain).

Many of us have spent decades assuming we are doing it wrong. We just aren't working hard enough. We haven't found the right diet or exercise program. We are lazy and gross, and we obviously have no willpower. We might notice a drop-dead gorgeous woman on one of those endless advertisements that flash before our eyes and think, *My God, what would it be like to look like that?* Then we assume if we simply add weight-training or take the newest supplement or start on the latest restrictive fad diet, our appearance (and obviously our lives) will improve. Our bodies might become like those images of the cultural ideal. The answer is out there. Somewhere. We know it! We just never can find it. And we spend years searching. Bending. Twisting. Counting. Lifting. Running. Restricting. Measuring. Injecting. Comparing. Criticizing. And absolutely *hating* our bodies for not being able to achieve perfection (then possibly giving up completely and downing ten golden Oreos in a spiral of shame).

After decades of imbibing ceaseless images of the cultural ideal and following the world's relentless "better-body" campaigns, we have fallen head over heels for what beauty culture and the wellness industry tell us about body types, aging, skin, cellulite, wrinkles, and the flab of our upper arms. It naturally follows, then, that even in middle age we can be confused about "normal" healthy human bodies. Our brains have bought wholeheartedly into the lie that our own beautifully ordinary, aging, perfectly normal bodies—these bodies that kept us safe into adulthood, these bodies that walked us down the aisle, these bodies that carried and birthed and nursed our precious babies, these bodies that make love to our spouse and hug a heartbroken friend and hike through the mountains and knead dough for Christmas morning cinnamon rolls—must not be *right*, somehow.

We believe the uniquely beautiful bodies God entrusted to each of us must not be *good* enough because we don't fit the cultural ideal for "beauty." And many of us continue to follow the stale breadcrumbs of generations before us, picking up body shame and various eating disorders like body dysmorphia, anorexia nervosa, bulimia nervosa, and binge eating disorder.

Digging Deeper into Eating Disorders and Body Shame[1]

- **Body dysmorphia** is an obsession with perceived (and often invisible) flaws in physical appearance that leads to repetitive behaviors like mirror checking, excessive grooming, skin picking, or repeated and compulsive comparison to the appearance of others that isn't explained by anorexia nervosa, bulimia, or another mood disorder such as depression or bipolar disorder.

- In **anorexia nervosa,** a restriction of daily calorie needs leads to significantly low body weight combined with an intense and overwhelming fear of becoming fat or gaining weight plus an inability to recognize the seriousness of a drastically low body weight.
- **Bulimia nervosa** involves recurrent episodes of binge eating that feel "out of control," followed by inappropriate behavior to compensate for the overeating that may include vomiting, use of laxatives or diuretic medications, fasting, or excessive exercise to prevent any weight gain.
- **Binge eating disorder** is defined by recurrent episodes of eating excessively large amounts of food in response to distressing emotions or stressors but without the compensatory behaviors found in bulimia nervosa.

With a lifetime prevalence in women of 9% (which is undoubtedly lower than the actual prevalence because many cases go unreported), we tend to believe that eating disorders are a problem for those in their teens and twenties.[2] We assume body-image issues are largely improved by the middle part of our lives, when we just want to eat "healthy." But in her book *The Wisdom of Your Body*, Dr. Hillary L. McBride, a licensed therapist who specializes in embodiment, points out that the damaging cycle of conditional self-worth and seeking external validation and affirmation based on our looks is ongoing, even into midlife and beyond:

A conditional self-worth and appearance-based value system is damaging wherever you are in life, but it becomes particularly problematic as we age. This is more true for women than for men, as there is a double standard in aging: aging men are seen as having increased prestige, whereas aging women have less importance as they are no longer seen as sex objects.[3]

Up to 75% of women of *all* ages (I'm raising my hand here) experience **disordered eating,** which involves food- and diet-related behaviors that don't quite meet the criteria for one of the above definitions of an eating disorder but still negatively affect our physical, mental, and emotional health.[4] The difference between disordered eating and an eating disorder is the severity, frequency, and impact our eating behaviors have on all the other aspects of our life. And unfortunately, these behaviors are often promoted by the "beauty and wellness" culture as "healthy"—hey, it's not a fad diet, it's a lifestyle!—with the hope that women will buy more books and exercise programs and smoothie recipes and dieting plans that promise to solve all our body issues (i.e., make us *thin*) and thus contribute to the still growing $4.4 trillion industry.

Disordered eating behaviors may include

- Avoiding entire food groups (ahem . . . carbs)
- Labeling foods as either "good" or "bad"
- Binge eating for celebration or wallowing or because for some reason you "deserve it"
- Attempting to "trick" yourself into feeling full with less food
- Fasting for weight loss
- Compensating for binging or eating a "forbidden" food through food restriction, exercise, or laxative use
- Following strict food rules or fad dieting (the keto diet, Whole 30, intermittent fasting, the caveman diet, the Adkins diet, the paleo diet . . . this list is endless)
- Constantly thinking about food and tracking food or calories to the point of preoccupation

- Checking your weight or measurements incessantly
- Feeling anxious, shameful, or guilty about simply eating food

Such behaviors may lead to weight loss in the short term (and may even be celebrated by diet and fitness culture); however, **weight cycling** (also termed yo-yoing) is almost always the ultimate result of disordered eating. We lose and gain and lose and gain all while making ourselves crazy with numbers and throwing our natural metabolism way out of whack. I think Elise Loehnen explains it best in her book *On Our Best Behavior: The Seven Deadly Sins and the Price Women Pay to Be Good*:

> Whenever I attempt deprivation, I can feel my body revolt, as though it's flipping me the middle finger by gaining a few pounds. It's asking for freedom from restraints and restrictions. It's asking me to allow that I have changed—and to love myself anyway.[5]

Deprivation of all kinds in the name of weight loss *will end*. But when we can stick with regular healthy and intuitive eating—which means enjoying a variety of foods from multiple food groups when we feel hungry then stopping when we feel full—rather than deprivation and restriction and the inevitable binge that follows, our bodies tend to have a **set weight point** where they will naturally settle.[6]

Retraining our thoughts and learning to detach from the beauty and wellness industry's relentless marketing toward a mostly unattainable (or at the very least fleeting) beauty ideal can take a lifetime. It begins with difficult self-reflection and endless self-compassion, and it may require support from a trained therapist, an eating disorder–informed provider, and/or a registered dietician. You are *more* than a body. And your health is *so much more* than your external appearance. Will you join me? Let's aim for something *better* than beautiful!

Focus on Healing

The more time I spend with other people—looking into their eyes, pressing my stethoscope gently against a frail chest, listening for the ins and outs of their breathing, noticing their hands gesture as they talk and imagining all the good hard work those hands have done, listening to people's stories—the more I can appreciate the beauty of the human form and *all* its ways. I'm convinced that it's the humanness, the uniqueness of each of God's creations, our common *humanity* that makes each one of us so breathtakingly beautiful. Truly, I can't think of anything more beautiful—more beloved, more treasured, more adored—than our individual bodies telling of God's unique love for every one of us.

The cultural ideal simply isn't God's design.

Our Creator made our form uniquely perfect and forever changing. Evolving. We begin young, fragile, and completely helpless, dependent upon others for survival but also able to withstand and grow and endure. Our beautiful bodies were *created* to adapt to whatever challenges we might face. Our bodies are meant to survive. And change. And if we're lucky enough, we age. The beautiful stories we survive and the breathtaking lives we live become etched across the bodies we inhabit, like cave drawings. Keeping tabs. Recording our woundedness with scars, our laughter with fine lines around the eyes, and our wisdom with white hair.

Despite what beauty and diet culture tells us, there is simply a vast and infinite array of different-appearing, uniquely perfect, and absolutely *normal* human bodies on this earth—of all shapes and sizes, skin colors, hair textures, muscle masses, eyes and noses, mouths and teeth, and curves and dents and leans. So, if you've been scrolling along and noticing thin, fit, clear-skinned and toned, predominantly white women with large, perky breasts and puffed lips and general firmness, and you find yourself looking down and around at your own body with its lines and marks and rolls and dimples and sagging breasts and general . . . well . . . looseness, wondering, *Is this right? Is my body supposed to look like this? Is this normal? Do other women's middle-aged bodies look like this?* the answer is probably yes. Yes, your body is supposed to look like this. Yes, you have the body of a middle-aged woman. Yes, my darling, you are perfectly normal. Yes, you are absolutely beautiful . . . and *more*!

If you don't believe me, please let my nineteen years of experience as a family practice physician with a fellowship in women's health (plus my very own midlife body) explain what I know about *normal*. The normal woman's body in midlife has

- A stretched and droopy belly button set atop silvery stretch marks lining a belly that may have carried a baby or two (or five) into the world.
- Two slightly mismatched breasts that hang a little lower and a little flatter over time, possibly after nursing all those babies. (Yes, most women hoist their flat pancakes up into a sports bra with a shove before heading to the gym.)
- Wider and fuller hips with a softer and wider waistline into our later thirties, then forties, then fifties. (Yep. Almost everyone has a flesh roll of one size or another when they sit. *Everyone.*)
- Brown age spots on our cheeks or hands and bright red hemangiomas dotting our chest or stomach and the occasional raised skin tag protruding from the slightly less elastic, increasingly wrinkled, and eventually crepe-papery skin of our neck.
- Darker and larger-appearing nipples plus darker and longer-appearing labia. (Mm-hmm. It's fine. I promise everyone's . . . umm . . . nether parts begin to look like that.)
- Decreasing muscle mass and increasing fat deposition with some amount of cellulite around our knees and hips and thighs.

- Coarser and thinner hair on our head with varying degrees of gray, acne along our jawline, and the occasional wiry hair on our chin (that can best be seen in the car's rearview mirror).

Normal is living in a forty- or fifty-year-old body that looks much different than our twenty- or thirty-year-old body. (I know. It seems they forgot to tell us about that between advertisements for anti-aging products shouting the promise of eternal youth.) And normal is simply embodying our beautifully aging form—the body that allows us to live all our days, a body that is forever precious and sexy and useful and functional, *a human body that is valuable, very much imperfect, and also perfectly normal!*

❊ ❊ ❊ ❊

When I took my daughter to the highly anticipated *Barbie* movie last summer for her seventh birthday, she wasn't terribly impressed since the movie was PG-13 and most of the humor went right over her head. But the other women in the theater all laughed at the same places alongside me. We all got it.

My favorite moment of the movie was a thirty-second clip toward the middle that stirred something deep inside me. Barbie has entered the Real World from Barbieland, and the reality of life is a shock to her system. She has never had real interactions with people or been mistreated or objectified in any way. She has never seen real life or anyone who isn't *perfect*. And in this particular scene she is sitting at a bus stop crying and wondering what she's supposed to do and how she's supposed to get out of this mess in the Real World and back to her perfect life, when she notices a woman sitting on the bench nearby wearing a cardigan and holding a bag on her lap with groceries or knitting tucked safely inside. The woman's face is worn and weathered, and her body is soft and full. She looks over at Barbie with concern. And in response Barbie, who has never laid eyes on a wrinkled face—the face of a good, hard, ordinary life well-lived—stops crying for a moment and wipes her tears. She stares for a moment, simply taking this woman in. Then she breaks into a wide smile and says, "You are *so* beautiful."

The elderly woman looks back unflinchingly at Barbie, and her eyes squinch into a smile that fills her whole face as she replies with love and confidence, "I know."[7]

That short clip was the theme of the whole movie, really. And I suppose it moved me so deeply because it is the theme of this whole book. Like most of us, I want to love my appearance (and of course, I would be lying if I said that I do not sometimes still long to be thin), but more than anything, I want to embrace the gift of what it means to be alive. *I want to be made well.*

I am happy to report I finally threw away those spirit-damaging, "weight-barometer" pre-pregnancy jeans, but it's only now—in my mid-forties—that my inner voice is beginning to speak to me gently. These days when I'm hungry for food or even just acceptance or love (which is usually all I'm ever really hungry for), my inner voice is beginning to respond tenderly, *Honey, eat if you're hungry. You deserve to eat when you're hungry. Food is good. Food is fuel for your body, and your body is good. Eat what sounds good to you. And maybe consider having something healthy along with every meal. An apple, perhaps. Apples are your favorite, right?*

Then, if in the middle of that internal conversation I accidentally pull down a sleeve of golden Oreos to numb myself from the current pain and anxiety of life by shoveling them into my mouth with a glass of milk, taking the time to open each one and lick out the sweet, white frosting, she simply smiles and says, *My darling, you are as loved and beautiful right now as you have ever been. I bet you'll feel better after a tall glass of water and a long walk. Hey, why don't you phone a friend?* And she's almost always right. It almost always helps.

I am *more* than a body. And my body's appearance is only one tiny facet of who I really am.

Though I fail at this more than I care to admit, I am learning, slowly, to *love* my body—her lines and wrinkles and scars, the beauty and lushness of her flesh and folds, the evidence of the heartachingly beautiful story of almost forty-five years to be seen here—and everything my body allows me to do. I am learning to trust my inner voice. I am learning to look into the mirror, deep into the eyes that haven't changed a bit over all these years, and I am learning to care for her the best way I know how. I am learning to peel off my swimsuit cover-up and waddle confidently to the pool so I can laugh and splash and cannonball off the side with my kids. I am learning to live with and truly love her—this body I *actually* have.

I am healing.

And I am finally learning to love my beautiful, God-given form.

Here are the best tips I can offer for your personal body-healing journey[8]

- Practice intuitive eating—eat and enjoy a variety of foods and stop eating when you feel full. Speak kindly to yourself. And rid yourself of any shame around food.

- Incorporate exercise into your daily way of life—something you enjoy, something that's easy, something that's fun, something you can do with a friend or with music in your ears—not for weight loss but for *health*. Exercise for your mental well-being and cardiovascular health and bone strength and to help you complete the stress cycle.

- Find supportive relationships and trusted healthcare professionals who will help you along the way (and remember to ditch body-shaming and diet-culture accounts on social media).

- Learn more about **body neutrality**—"a state of accepting and respecting your body as it is, prioritizing how you feel and what you do, rather than how you look."[9]

- Set boundaries with people or experiences that may be triggering or shaming for you.
- Be gentle with yourself.
- Believe you are beautiful . . . because you are!

Let's not wait even a moment more. Let's not believe the noise. Let's not buy into beauty and diet culture and the ridiculous lie of "ideal." Instead, let's accept ourselves as beautiful and worthy and treasured and adored. Us—in *these* bodies, at *this* weight, with *these* imperfections, with *these* faces—simply living our good, hard, ordinary lives. Beautiful then, beautiful now. Not next week or next month. Not when we lose those last ten (or twenty or fifty) pounds. Not with Botox or perkier breasts or more fashionable clothes or firmer thighs. Not one day years from now, looking back at old photos and noticing how beautiful we *used* to be. But today. Just like this.

Beauty isn't something *out there* for you to find. It isn't something for you to chase or buy or inject with Botox or cover or squeeze into Spanx or starve or attempt to cleanse or shame away. And it isn't something for you to struggle after and strive for and yearn toward. No. It's just here. Beauty is *in* you. It has been in you all along because you were made by His design. Beauty *IS* you. You are so beautiful. *You.* Your life, your face, your shape, your wrinkles, your spirit, and your horrible and tortuous, mesmerizing and ordinary, breathtaking and miraculous story. You are *more* than beautiful.

And I am, too. Now I can honestly say, "I know."

9

GENERALIZED ANXIETY, DEPRESSION, AND OTHER MOOD DISORDERS

We had an earthquake in Utah during the first week of school shutdown and the shelter-in-place order at the beginning of the coronavirus pandemic.

I clicked away at the computer keys in the early-morning darkness of my office—savoring the part of the day reserved just for me and hoping some quiet time with my thoughts at the computer might ease the anxiety I'd been carrying about remote learning with five kids and the general uneasiness of the world—when suddenly the room began to rumble and shake. It's amazing how a brain can process things in nanoseconds, isn't it? *This is an earthquake!? What do I do in an earthquake? Oh, right! Cover my head! Find a doorway!*

I made my way to the door frame and gripped the molding just in time to see the chandelier swinging wildly like a pendulum back and forth above our worn kitchen table. The jerking intensified, and glass shattered throughout the house as frames vaulted from their picture ledges and round-bottomed mugs in the kitchen toppled from their shelves.

Cries of "Moommmyyyy!" emerged from the bedrooms upstairs, which sent me crawling on my hands and knees up the chattering stairs to reach them.

"Everyone get outside! Grab your shoes and get your glasses! Outside, now!" I barked like a drill sergeant, positive we had just entered apocalyptic territory. Everyone would need their eyes and feet to survive! Two minutes of quaking can seem like an eternity, and apparently a 5.7 on the Richter scale feels like the walls of a home will topple at any moment. But then just as quickly as it began, the shaking stopped.

I felt rattled to my core. *First a global pandemic with rising death counts, overflowing intensive care unit (ICU) beds, and empty grocery store shelves. Plus, strained family relationships and unsubstantiated finger-pointing and hateful political vitriol everywhere I turned. Now this? An earthquake??? Were we truly experiencing the end times?* We felt aftershocks all day, some as high as 2.4 on the scale. They came frequently enough that my children would simply look up from their Zoom screens to call out, "Do you feel that?" or "Yep. I think it's another one. Moooom, it's another one!" before returning to their remote learning assignments.

My middle schooler had an orthodontist appointment that afternoon, and as the chandelier swayed once again over the kitchen table, I ordered everyone to the car.

"What? Why do *we* have to go? I have class! I can't miss this Zoom. Mom, why can't we just stay home? I'll watch the little kids while you take him. Mom, come on. Whyyyy?" my oldest argued.

"Because if this is really the end of the world, we are going to be TOGETHER for it!" I shot back. If I'd been a marsupial, say a koala with a roomy-enough pouch attached to my body, I would've been tucking my children safely inside. Forever. I never wanted to leave them again.

And it wasn't too long after that day that I suffered my first full-blown panic attack.

I lay down like I always do after my normal nightly routine—brushing, double-checking my phone alarm for the morning, snapping my night mouth guard for teeth grinding into place, arranging the covers far away from my claustrophobic feet, then reaching my arm across the king-sized divide to gently find my husband's arm. When we were newly married, I slept with my leg slung over his waist as we spooned together, always touching. But now, I long for space to stretch out. Untouched.

On this particular night, instead of settling into silent prayer as I closed my eyes ready for sleep, intense panic hurled me into a frenzy like an unexpected 5.7-on-the-Richter-scale earthquake. BAM! My heart began to pound, heavy and hard. Racing away and skipping a few beats. My head buzzed and swirled with every thought I'd had for the last month as my body began to drip with sweat. It really did feel just like the textbooks describe. *Oh, this is exactly what it means to feel "impending doom."* Because if I didn't get out of that bed, out of that room, out of my swirling mind, I was sure the world might open from the center and swallow me whole. Or at any rate, I might possibly die.

I gulped for air, grabbed my pillow, and headed for the living room. I paced across the cream and gray Bohemian rug spread on the floor, back and forth. Breathing long and slow, I pressed my hand to my chest, exhaled through pursed lips, and prayed: *Jesus be near, Jesus be near, Jesus be near.* The change of venue helped a little, along with the pacing and breathing and chanting in prayer. And eventually with my heart still palpable beneath my palm, I was able to quiet my mind before settling into sleep on the couch.

I wasn't positive it was a panic attack (thinking maybe it was a premature hot flash?) until it happened again a few weeks later at four in the morning when my daughter came in to wake me in her rumpled, middle-of-the-night kind of way.

"Momma, will you come snuggle me?"

I shuffled after her and settled myself beside her in that little twin bed with the pink floral quilt from Target. Nothing felt out of the ordinary as her night-light cast bluish-green stars across the ceiling, and I fell asleep to the gentle in-and-out of her quiet breath, inhaling the sweet lavender scent left over from her evening bath.

After dozing for an hour or so, I woke with a start. Suddenly wide awake. Suddenly hyper-aware of time passing. Of my children growing. Of my life changing—the end of one chapter and a new one beginning. Questions began pelting my brain like fierce, tiny daggers. *What are you doing with your one precious, beautiful life? Where are you going? What happens next? What if the world ends? And what is the point?* I leapt out of bed toward the living room, where I began pacing once again.

Turns out, my anxiety is always *right there*, waiting to pounce.

I thought I'd have more figured out by my forties. I thought I'd feel more settled as a wife and a mother and more confident in my career and within my close family and friend relationships. I thought I'd have more peace and clarity in my faith and religion, about my body, my purpose, my life. And in some ways, I do. But then these subtle and seismic shifts arise to shake things up and sift the contents of my life through the proverbial strainer:

What's important?

What matters?

What can be let go of? Or put away?

Is this serving my life right now or the cause of far too much anxiety?

Is it helping? Or hurting?

Is this simply too heavy to carry forward?

Can I put another thing down?

Sometimes we feel the magnitude of two tectonic plates pushing and grinding against each other—a child grows into a new stage or encounters a new future-altering dilemma, our husband is up for a promotion at work that may or may not be in the family's best interest, an unforeseen stress fracture disrupts a once-stable extended family relationship, another school shooting threatens our children's safety and our peace of mind, a war breaks out overseas, or a global pandemic divides our nation in two. And other times, the change is almost imperceptible—like another pair of shoes outgrown or giant Chiclet teeth slowly edging into place or one inch higher ticked on the wall. Just when I get a few details ironed out and find my footing on solid ground, a life issue arises like an aftershock, leaving me unsteady and swaying as the floor beneath my feet rumbles and the walls seem ready to topple at any moment. Time and again, I find myself grabbing for a door frame to steady myself or crawling on my hands and knees to safety.

My anxiety during Covid shutdown and the earthquake and attempting to navigate online learning with my growing children mixed with all the stress of raising teenagers and my changing forty-plus-year-old body grew absolutely paralyzing. It was enough that on one particularly tense morning my husband said gently (and possibly with his own fear and trembling), "Honey, would it be okay if I reached out to someone?"

"What do you mean?" I said, annoyed.

"Can I call this friend of mine at work to see if she can see you? Maybe you should talk to someone."

"Is it *really* that bad?" I thought I was managing okay. Or okay enough anyway. I thought I was hiding the chaos and constant anxiety of my insides. I thought I played a good game. I thought I put on a good show. But . . . no.

"It's getting really bad, hon. I hate seeing you like this."

Huh. Apparently, my anxiety was enough that my physician-husband used his VIP pass at the university hospital where he works to phone a physician friend and get me on her schedule for the *following day*. It couldn't wait another week, another month, another six months of suffering. For any of us.

And the following day when I poured my problems out to this incredibly kind doctor, I said something like, "Well, I'm having panic attacks, and my periods are terrible. Plus, in the five or so days leading up to my period, I'm not anywhere close to myself. I feel . . . well . . . insane, basically. I get so revved up! I'm angry a lot, and I snap at the kids too much. But then other mornings, I can barely get out of bed. I can't sleep at night. I can't think straight during the day. And I'm just not . . . me. It's so much more than just stress."

Except I wanted to explain it all away.

"But really, I'm fine. I'll be okay. It's not that big a deal. I'm just a little anxious sometimes. And it could be so much worse. Other people have it so much worse! I guess maybe we should check my thyroid."

But something needed to change.

After a full physical followed by normal laboratory work (where, yes, shockingly my thyroid function was normal) and a trial of one medication that didn't seem to help, I followed up six weeks later and together we discovered an answer.

I've found countless indispensable tools for my journey along this winding path of life—good friends, constant prayer, warm baths at the end of a long day, books and stories and words, a few of my favorite podcasts in my ears, long walks with my dog, Fern, or our sweet kitty purring at my feet. I tuck each of these tools into my back pocket for safe keeping just like my kids when they happen upon a tiny treasure on our mountain hikes. Except instead of sticks or rocks or fossils or "the beautifulest leaf ever," the most important tool I've collected these last few years is my morning Lexapro.

✳ ✳ ✳ ✳

If you came to me as a patient and described almost daily head-aches with the occasional debilitating monthly migraine layered on top. Plus, chronic neck and shoulder pain so intense it causes numbness and tingling into your fingertips. And now the newly acquired thunderclap of dread from an occasional panic attack that leaves you breathless and panting . . .

Or if you admitted that when one of your loved ones leans in for a kiss goodbye before leaving for work or heading out with friends or out of town for a soccer tournament, an immediate thought comes barreling in . . . *What if this is the last time? What if this is it? What if this kiss goodbye really is goodbye? Forever?* And then morbid images of that loved one in a fiery crash sitting lifeless in the front seat, bruised and bloody, repeatedly flash before your eyes . . .

Or if you reported nights of insomnia spent pacing the floor while your heart races or frequently pulling a pillow and blanket down to the couch hoping to find sleep with a change of venue. Or crippling anxiety when doing normal adult things like driving to work or finding a new address or making a few important phone calls or buying a plane ticket or switching your utility bill after a move. You know, typical, run-of-the-mill adult stuff . . .

I would listen intently, take notice of your fidgeting hands, jot down a few notes, ask thoughtful questions about exercise and sleep hygiene and herbal supplements and alcohol use and support systems from family and friends, and administer a couple of questionnaires as diagnostic tools. Then I would begin to use the working diagnosis of generalized anxiety disorder before tenderly discussing all the treatment options such as cognitive behavioral therapy and a trial of a selective serotonin reuptake inhibitor (SSRI).

Like the one that works for me: Lexapro.

And when you protested—"But my life is so good! I'm fine. Really. I have absolutely nothing to be anxious about"—I would reassure you that's why we call it generalized anxiety *disorder*. This type of anxiety is not merely a normal response to the occasional life stressor or a normal grief reaction following one of life's inevitable tragedies. And it's more than simply hormonal fluctuations

148

that cause PMS symptoms or even PMDD for a few days before your period. It's a chemical imbalance of the brain. A mix of both genetics and environmental factors swirled together and largely out of your control. *A disorder*. Generalized anxiety disorder.

Having normal mental health means displaying a range of feelings—happy, sad, angry, disappointed, overjoyed—that are appropriate to the current situation. We can't just feel happy all the time! But sometimes the normal feelings that are perfectly appropriate for a given situation become something much *more*.

Digging Deeper into Mood Disorders

Generalized anxiety disorder (GAD) is excessive worry that invades multiple aspects of life—worry about your kids, your relationships, your health, your work or career path, your pets, your house, and your daily life events. It's a worry that feels completely uncontrollable and causes significant distress (i.e., disaster) that persists daily over a six-month period or more.

GAD is one of the most common mood disorders with a lifetime prevalence of 5–12%, which means more than one in ten people will experience GAD in their lifetime. It's twice as common in females and often diagnosed around age thirty in those who've had a tendency toward anxious traits during their growing-up years. We know underlying genetics *and* environmental factors play a role.[1]

Here's what we look for to make a diagnosis of anxiety[2]

- Excessive worry that occurs on most days over six months
- Worry that is difficult to control
- Plus, three or more of these symptoms
  - Restlessness
  - Fatigue
  - Poor concentration
  - Irritability

- Muscle tension (which may manifest as a stiff neck and shoulders or regular migraine headaches)
- Other physical complaints (termed **somatic symptoms**) such as stomach pain or changes in bowel habits, irregular heartbeat, chest pain, or dizziness
- Trouble with sleep
- Worry that causes problems in daily functioning
- Worry that is not due to other illness such as hyperthyroidism, substance use, or another mood disorder

The GAD-7 is a tool medical providers use to both rate symptoms as mild, moderate, or severe and assess the response to the various treatment options that we will be discussing in more detail below. You can find a complete GAD-7 in appendix 1.

❊ ❊ ❊ ❊

Now, let's move on to **depression**. Feeling "depressed" is a common way we describe our moments of sadness or despair, our occasional discouragement or fleeting feelings of hopelessness, our tearfulness, or even the numbness we feel following a life tragedy that knocks us off our feet. We may even say flippantly to a friend after a particularly hard day, "I'm so depressed." But **major depressive disorder** is *more* than feeling down; it's a profound sadness that settles in and won't go away.

We think of depression as a problem of the brain, but really, depression can affect many organ systems and multiple aspects of our lives, including our day-to-day emotions, our sleep and appetite, our relationships, our thought patterns, our overall physical health, and other chronic illnesses.

Major depressive disorder tops the list as the most common mood disorder. Nearly 20% of Americans will experience an episode of depression in their lifetime. Furthermore, depression can be increasingly common for women with age, perhaps due to the hormonal chaos of declining estrogen during perimenopause since estrogen works to boost **serotonin**, a neurotransmitter that is partly responsible for our mood. Other risk factors for developing depression include a family history of depression and other mood disorders, a history of adverse childhood experiences (or ACEs) as we discussed in chapter 3, socioeconomic factors and financial hardships, poor sleep, smoking and substance abuse, life stressors, poor social support/connections, and other chronic medical illness.[3]

Here's what we look for to make a diagnosis of depression[4]

- Five or more depressive symptoms are present every day for two weeks in a row:
  - Depressed mood
  - Loss of interest or pleasure in most activities
  - Weight loss or weight gain due to changes in appetite
  - Inability to sleep or sleeping *all* the time
  - Changes in activity level—either feeling overly agitated or moving *extremely* slow as if underwater
  - Daily fatigue
  - Feelings of worthlessness or excessive guilt
  - Decreased concentration or indecisiveness
  - Recurrent thoughts of death or suicidal thoughts/plans.
- Symptoms cause problems at work, home, and in other areas of daily life.
- Symptoms can't be attributed to substance abuse, medications/herbal supplements, or some other medical illness.
- Symptoms can't be explained by another mood disorder such as **bipolar disorder** in which similar depressive symptoms alternate with episodes of mania (characterized by extreme elevations in mood, emotions, energy, and activity level) or **substance-induced mood disorder** in which

symptoms occur as a consequence of alcohol, prescription medication, or illicit drug use/abuse.

Two patient health questionnaires (the PHQ-2 and PHQ-9) are used by medical providers to first screen and then evaluate symptoms of depression, which are then rated as mild, moderate, or severe.

You can find the full depression screening questionnaire, the PHQ-9, in appendix 3. Here is the shortened version, called the PHQ-2, which is often used as a quick screening tool during preventative healthcare maintenance exams:[5]

Short Patient Health Questionnaire (PHQ-2)

Name:		Date:			
Over the past 2 weeks, how often have you been bothered by any of the following problems?	Not at all	Several days	More than half the days	Nearly every day	Total point score:
Little interest or pleasure in doing things?	0	1	2	3	
Feeling down, depressed, or hopeless?	0	1	2	3	
	___	+ ___	+ ___	+ ___	___

Score interpretation:		
PHQ-2 score	Probability of major depressive disorder (%)	Probability of any depressive disorder (%)
1	15.4	36.9
2	21.1	48.3
3	38.4	75.0
4	45.5	81.2
5	56.4	84.6
6	78.6	92.9

There are other forms of depression that may not fit the definition of major depressive disorder. **Dysthymia**, also termed **persistent depressive disorder,** is a milder, longer-lasting form of depression in which three or more depressive symptoms—specifically including depressed mood—persist for two consecutive years.[6] And **seasonal affective disorder (SAD)** is an episodic form of depression that occurs during certain times of the year—typically from late fall to early spring—and tends to recur annually.[7]

Severe depression may include thoughts or plans for suicide or harming others, symptoms of psychosis such as delusions or hallucinations, and impairment in basic everyday functioning. In severe cases, hospitalization may be necessary to intervene and initiate immediate treatment. If you ever feel like you might hurt yourself or others, there is help available to you. Call 911, contact your doctor or nurse, go to the emergency department, or contact the 988 Suicide & Crisis lifeline by texting 988, calling 988, or going to www.988lifeline.org/chat online. Don't wait. Reach out for help right away.

Any combination of the above disorders can lead to a decreased quality of life or decreased enjoyment in our daily life, a higher risk of suicide, negative outcomes of other medical disorders, and a higher risk for death. Plus, our mental well-being affects the loved ones we spend time with every day.

Many treatment options are available, and none of us must suffer through anxiety or depression or other mood disorders alone.

Treatment of various mood disorders depends on a few factors

- The unique and specific set of symptoms
- Each medication's safety profile and possible side effects
- Other medical illnesses including the other medications you take and any possible interactions
- Cost
- Any previous treatment for mood disorders and previous response to such treatment
- And, most importantly, your personal preferences as a patient

In general, treatment for generalized anxiety, major depressive disorder, dysthymia, or seasonal affective disorder begins with an antidepressant medication *and* therapy, which have been proven to be more effective in combination than either of these treatments alone. The antidepressant medications are grouped into classes depending on how they work in the brain.

These are the most used medications for mood disorders

- Selective serotonin reuptake inhibitors (SSRIs) like Lexapro, Celexa, Paxil, Prozac, and Zoloft
- Serotonin-norepinephrine reuptake inhibitors (SNRIs) like Effexor or Cymbalta
- Atypical antidepressants like Wellbutrin or Remeron
- Serotonin modulators like Trazadone

Typically, SSRIs provide the most benefit with the least amount of risk and are a good place to start for treating mood disorders. Side effects may include nausea, jitteriness, changes in sleep, weight gain, headaches, and sexual side effects. Side effects of these medications tend to be dose dependent (meaning risk for side effects increases with increasing doses) and may improve or go away completely after you've been on the medication for a while.[8] For SSRIs, the sexual side effects of decreased libido and difficulty achieving orgasm are the primary reasons people stop taking the medication and try something else. The group of atypical antidepressants, like Wellbutrin, tend to not affect sexual function.

Along with medication, going to therapy can help with coping skills and improve adaptive ways of thinking about problems. In addition, the use of relaxation techniques, a healthy diet, adequate sleep, social connection, and regular daily exercise may improve mood symptoms.[9]

For anyone with symptoms of mania, which may be part of mixed symptom depression or bipolar disorder as mentioned above, SSRIs and similar medications may worsen those symptoms. Be sure to tell your doctor if you notice an oddly elevated mood, emotions, or energy/activity level on SSRI medication or other medications prescribed for mood disorders.

In general, treatment may begin to help with symptoms within two weeks; however, it can take up to twelve weeks to see the full effect. If after this time symptoms are not improved, options for changes to the treatment plan include increasing the dose, adding an additional medication, switching to a new class of medication, or taking another step like more intensive therapy.

Focus on Healing

I would never respond to the very real issues a patient shares in clinic with even an ounce of shame. I would not call *any* of those very real issues a lack of self-control or a weakness in character or some deficit of faith. But I'm sorry to admit that's exactly how I responded to myself when I started medication for generalized anxiety.

I spent years—a decade, maybe—ignoring the fact that I popped Tylenol or Ibuprofen like breath mints to treat daily headaches, ignoring the debilitating monthly migraine layered on top that sent me to bed for twenty-four hours (and simply blaming PMS), ignoring the chronic nagging muscle soreness in my neck and back from the hard, stiff knots that drew my shoulders up to my ears, ignoring the interrupted sleep and resulting chronic daily fatigue, ignoring that although I managed to navigate a husband and five children, a medical degree and part-time career, the running of an entire household, plus the one million things I must attend to every week, sometimes the idea of doing very basic adult things like finding a new address or making a few hard phone calls or buying a plane ticket sent me into a tailspin of anxiety and dread.

I spent years ignoring *all* of it.

I attributed my symptoms to life. I blamed hormones. I made endless excuses: *I just need to exercise more! I just need to eat better! I just need to get off social media, organize my house, lose a few pounds, get out in nature, drink more water, take a power nap, practice yoga, and focus on self-care! I just need to get my act together! Get my life together!* I didn't have anxiety, I was fine. *I am FINE*, I'd say.

Of course, for my friends or my patients or my neighbors or for the other moms in playgroup or anyone else who might recount any combination of similar debilitating symptoms, I recommended therapy and a trial of an SSRI. I encouraged it, prescribed it, applauded it. But medication to treat anxiety for *myself*? Nah.

Instead, my internal voice began its typical barrage of criticism: *What is WRONG with you? Pull it together! You have a million things to be grateful for. So many other people in this world have it entirely worse than you. You're weak. Plus, it's probably just your hormones. You'll get through it. It will get better. Maybe next month. Maybe when the kids are all in school. Maybe when you figure out what you're doing in your career. Maybe once you start exercising regularly again. Maybe if you could just get rid of those last fifteen pounds. Taking medication for "anxiety" is such an obvious sign of your failure. You can do this on your own—just work harder! You are supposed to be the helper . . . how dare you EVER admit you need help.*

Turns out, I am quite accomplished at really seeing and noticing *other people*—their goodness, their love, their gifts, their belovedness. In fact, sometimes when I'm examining the in and out of a patient's lungs or walking along beside a friend on the path near my house just listening while she relays a recent life struggle, I imagine how God looks at them. Loves them. And adores them. Compassion researcher Kristin Neff defines this as compassion—the ability to recognize suffering, flaws, and fragility as part of this shared human condition. When I'm with patients, I'm reminded with such assuredness that each beautiful human was made with deep, abiding love *on purpose.* And each person's life has a great depth of meaning. They are a treasure to be adored! But then in the very next breath, I might turn and speak hatred to myself.

I am full of compassion for others, but I am not always so good at speaking that same voice of love and care for myself. It's the *self*-compassion I am working on these days. Neff goes on to describe self-compassion in a way I certainly need to hear:

> Self-compassion involves wanting health and well-being for oneself and leads to proactive behavior to better one's situation, rather than passivity. And self-compassion doesn't mean that I think my problems are more important than yours, it just means I think that my problems are *also* important and worthy of being attended to. . . . Self-compassion is . . . giving ourselves unconditional kindness and comfort while embracing the human experience.[10]

So, what about you? Did anything in this chapter on anxiety or depression strike a chord? If so, could you swallow down your pride, shush that minimizing inner critic, embrace every ounce of self-compassion you can muster, then be proactive by making an appointment with your primary medical provider to discuss your mood and treatment options a little further? More than anything I want to tell you it's normal to feel up and down. It's actually healthy to have feelings that fit your current situation. But if those sad or anxious feelings settle in and become *more* than that, it's okay to get help.

For me, practicing self-compassion begins by swallowing a small white pill every morning along with regular therapy. And honestly, it's making all the difference.

10

SEX AND SLEEP

Bringing Sexy Back in Your (continuous positive airway pressure) CPAP Machine

"Hey! How are you?" my friend Emily asked brightly, scootching down the bleachers to make room.

I settled myself wearily beside her for our boys' Saturday morning basketball game and gave her the common response, "Ugh. Tired. Why are these games so *early*?"

My daughter interrupted our conversation to hound me for an old, squished-up granola bar from my purse (because of course we hadn't had time for breakfast before we left the house). Then she ran off to play with her friends in the hall as I continued, "Anyway, how are *you*?"

Emily laughed. "You know, I can honestly say I'm less tired now that I started using a CPAP machine. Isn't that crazy? I'm only 42, and I have sleep apnea! I went to my doctor a few months ago because I was so tired. Like, *all the time* tired. We did a bunch of blood work, then I ended up doing a sleep study because she asked me if I snore. I can't believe the difference this stupid CPAP is making after only two months!"

"Oh, I bet! I wish my husband would go for a sleep study. He snores like crazy."

"Yeah. Maybe this is weird to share and totally TMI, but now I'm struggling to feel sexy with a CPAP strapped to my face. Especially when I slip it over my nose while we cuddle, you know . . . *afterward*." She rolled her eyes.

We both laughed a little, then I replied, "I can totally understand that. Not weird at all."

I told her about my friend Amy, who recently posted a selfie together with her husband in twin nasal CPAP masks at bedtime with the caption, "Bringing sexy back with our his-and-hers CPAP machines!"[1] Then we dove into a whole conversation about sex and midlife and our chubby bodies and kid-stress and sleep (or lack thereof) because I have never been the type of person for idle conversation. Basketball game or not. Tired or not. New friends, old friends, barely friends, or some kid's mom I just met, please bring *all* your hard topics to any conversation you have with me so we can *really* get to the good stuff!

Digging Deeper into Sleep

Sleep is tricky, isn't it? We know sleep is important and necessary for good health and daytime productivity and ongoing learning and bodily healing. But then, most nights we stay up way too late binge-watching the latest series on Hulu even though we know we need to get up early the next morning. Or, worse, we scroll. Our thumbs begin flicking, and we laugh or fume at the things we see flashing before our eyes. Or sometimes, miraculously, we do manage to lay our exhausted bodies down in bed at a reasonable time, hoping to get enough sleep for that big thing tomorrow morning, but instead of settling in, our minds click on in a frenzy.

We think about the kids. We think about everything we need to do tomorrow. We think about all the things we didn't get done today. We think about our weight and those cookies we ate after dinner. We think about what our mother said the last time we called. We think about our childhood hurts. We think about re-modeling the living room. We think about what we're going to wear to that special event next month. We think about God's existence. We think about the flab collecting in a roll around our middle. We think about doing more sit-ups. We think about whether or not our kids have any friends. We think about the next series on Hulu that we can barely wait for (it's coming out next week!). We think about how long it's been since we've had sex. We think about how quickly time is passing. We think about school shootings. We think about dinners for the rest of the week. And mostly, we think about how we should be sleeping.

When our weary heads hit the pillow, we hop on the dreaded hamster wheel and run headlong into thinking about *all the things*, and once the speed of the wheel kicks in and our little brains begin pumping, we know it's over. Sleep definitely won't come. At least not anytime soon. Then when we wake up the next morning, we are *so tired*. In a fog, we immediately vow that tonight things will be different. No Hulu. No scrolling. No hamster wheel. Because, ugh. We need to get more sleep!

Maybe it's different for you.

Maybe you stay up late because you have a whole slew of teenagers living in your home (honestly, just one or two teen-agers can feel like a whole slew) who are out until midnight on the weekends, and you can't really fall asleep until everyone is tucked safely into their beds. Or maybe your darling little daugh-ter who is seven years old and clearly capable of staying in her room for the night still tiptoes up to your bed on occasion and whispers, "Momma, can you come snuggle me?" And you do be-cause she is the youngest (and we tend to do lots of things we said we'd never do with the youngest). Or maybe your hamster wheel doesn't begin turning until you jerk awake at three in the morning, panting and sweating. Or maybe you have a very sweet spouse who also very *un*-sweetly happens to rattle the rafters with his foghorn snoring, which makes it almost impossible to fall back to sleep.

Or wait, maybe it's *you* who is snoring! Are you getting plenty of sleep but still walking around tired throughout the day? Does your bed partner ever mention you appear to stop breathing during the night, or do you frequently wake with a choking sensation? It's possible you may need an evaluation for sleep apnea like my friend Emily.

Sleep apnea is caused by airway obstruction during the night and can result in excessive daytime sleepiness. It is generally more common in men but can increase for women in midlife, especially for those with a history of high blood pressure, obesity, and a large neck and/or waist circumference. These days, the evaluation for sleep apnea begins with a device that can be worn at home so it's super easy, and you'll only need the formal overnight sleep study if the initial test is abnormal. Several treatment options for sleep apnea are available and may include the use of a continuous positive airway pressure (CPAP) machine.[2]

Whatever the (often multiple and compounded) reasons— kids or stress or scrolling or snoring or sleep apnea—sleep may worsen in midlife. The areas of the brain that regulate sleep and set our circadian rhythms are heavily influenced by estrogen and progesterone, and fluctuations in these hormones during peri-menopause may affect what used to be normal sleep patterns. Add to that the increasing number of complicating factors like hot flashes, teenagers, the stress of caregiver roles, a changing and aging body that may have underlying chronic illness, plus a changing and aging spouse who may snore (possibly from sleep apnea), or conditions such as **restless leg syndrome** (RSL), which causes an uncontrollable urge to move your legs that tends to worsen in the evening hours, or **periodic limb movement disorder** (PLMD), which causes jerking, cramping, or twisting of your legs during sleep. Whatever the reason—whether it's difficulty falling to sleep at night, staying asleep throughout the night, or frequent very early morning waking—for 40–60% of women in midlife, sleep is just tricky.[3]

Many effective treatment options are available for all types of insomnia, including over-the-counter (OTC) medications, prescription medications, and dietary supplementation with melatonin. Please note that *all* the treatments used for sleep problems must be used with caution as they share a similar risk of side effects like decreased alertness, motor incoordination, and next-day sleepiness. Furthermore, these treatments can be habit-forming, and for some, regular use of medications for sleep may worsen depressive symptoms or suicidal ideation. Finally, a select few who use sleep-aid medications may even experience bizarre behaviors like hallucinations, agitation, sleepwalking episodes, and attempts to do daytime activities like driving, eating, or sex while fully asleep.[4]

Medications and supplements used to treat sleep issues should always be used *together with* improved bedtime practices and therapy. We'll talk more about ways to improve your sleep hygiene to get better rest later in this chapter. As always, your healthcare provider is the best source of information for further questions and concerns related to sleep and may recommend a referral to a sleep specialist for a more in-depth evaluation and treatment.

Now, Let's Talk about Sex

Like sleep, sex can be pretty tricky too, can't it? We wonder, *Are we having enough? Are we enjoying it? Do we want more? Or less? Can we even find the time for it in the middle of our busy lives? Are our spouses happy with the sex we do have? Are we disappointing them? Are we disappointing us? Who, exactly, decided what is the "normal and expected" number of times per week a couple should have sex? (Probably men.) And is anyone having the kind of sex after twenty years of marriage that looks*

*like what we see portrayed in the media? Are we normal? Am I
... normal?*

I've always wondered why men and women are made so . . .
differently. Men are generally pleased with the act of intercourse—
stimulation through sex obviously happens in all the right areas
resulting in orgasm with ejaculation. And for the most part, men
desire sex with their partner in order to *feel* connected. If we've
been passing like ships through the night, interacting via text during the day, shlepping one kid here and another kid there with
barely a peck on the lips in the morning, my husband craves sex
so we can feel like a connected and in-sync married couple again.

Somehow, I'm wired in reverse. Women generally prefer a close
connection with our partner *before* sex can sound enticing. We
want to feel seen and heard and understood and known. We tend
to think, *But we've been passing like ships through the night and
interacting via text throughout the day and shlepping kids back
and forth . . . shouldn't we, you know, CONNECT first before
stripping off our clothes?*

Plus, women often cannot achieve orgasm without external,
non-penetrative stimulation of the clitoris. For most women, a
little extra care for an average of over thirteen minutes (yes, studies show a mean of *13.4 minutes* . . . over twice as long as men)
must be taken to stimulate *exactly* the right areas to achieve orgasm.[5] Many women in typical heterosexual relationships (myself included) may grow frustrated by these anatomic differences
between men and women, thinking, *Is this taking too long? Am I
taking too long? Is he bored? How long will he wait? Should we
simply . . . move on? Is there something wrong with me? With
him? With us? Is sex frustrating for other couples?* Then when I
voice my concerns about the added time and extra care required,
my husband says something like, "Are you kidding me? I enjoy the
wait! I absolutely *love* doing that with you! Honey, when *you're*
satisfied it makes sex that much better for *me*, too." And I wonder
(again) why I worry at all.

Difficulties related to sex in midlife and perimenopause are based on a whole variety of factors that can be summed up as

1. Complicated
2. Unique to every individual person and every individual couple
3. Influenced by *all the other issues* in our lives

Sexual dysfunction is a sexual problem that is persistent or recurrent and causes marked personal distress or difficulty in relationships. Problems with sex can range from lack of sexual desire, impaired ability to achieve orgasm, pain with sexual activity, or a combination of all these issues. Such difficulties are typically multifactorial and may increase during midlife because of decreased sensation/innervation of the clitoris or vaginal dryness (termed **genitourinary symptoms of perimenopause** or **GSM**),[6] medication side effects (these may include antidepressants, beta blockers, spironolactone, opioids, and trazadone), other chronic medical conditions such as diabetes, depression, or high blood pressure to name a few, lack of communication or closeness with a partner, or an increase in the general stressors of life.

Remember that hamster wheel that keeps us from sleeping? I know I tend to hop on my hamster wheel of anxiety riiiiiiiight at the beginning of foreplay, and I must continually bring my mind back to the matter at hand (sex and the clitoris!). Can you relate? That dreaded wheel makes it awfully hard to concentrate on the good stuff, right? Plus, what about the slew of teenagers? The interrupting seven-year-old? The never-ending to-do list? Our bone-aching tiredness? We *want* to want to have a healthy and active sex life with our loving partner. But sometimes good, hard, ordinary life can wreak havoc on desire.

Desire can mean either *actively* wanting to engage in sexual activity or *being receptive* to engaging in sexual activity. The latter is called **responsive desire**, meaning we choose physical intimacy for comfort or satisfying a partner or growing closer in a relationship. And in this perfectly normal form of desire, physical arousal comes *after* the decision to have a sexual interaction with our partner. In this scenario, foreplay with an engaged and patient partner plays an essential role in getting us to the arousal part.

Sometimes, we simply get bored after being in a relationship for a while. Honest discussions with our partner about trying new things may improve connection and intimacy. Things like spending a night away from home, trying a new sexual position, incorporating a vibrator device for increased clitoral stimulation, or having sex in a different location or at a different time of the day might all help to liven things up. Establishing a regular date night, even if only once a month, tends to improve sexual satisfaction for couples. Date night is a time and place to hash out all the thoughts from the hamster wheel and enjoy connection *outside* the bedroom (which typically means things will improve sexually back in the bedroom!).

When both active and responsive desire are lacking, **sexual interest/arousal disorder** (**SIAD**) may be the cause, and it's diagnosed when three of the following symptoms are present for six months *and* cause significant personal distress or interpersonal difficulty:[7]

- Reduced/absent desire for sex
- Reduced/absent sexual thoughts
- Reduced/absent receptivity of sexual activity
- Reduced/absent sexual pleasure
- Reduced/absent desire triggered by sexual stimulation
- Reduced/absent genital sensations

Your healthcare provider is the best source of information for questions and concerns related to your symptoms of sexual dysfunction. Talk with your provider about the medication you are taking and whether side effects from those medications may be contributing to your symptoms. Work together with your provider to rule out other medical conditions such as depression or fatigue due to sleep apnea because the desire for sex can be affected by these and other chronic conditions. Know that prescription medications may be moderately effective in treating SIAD. And understand that satisfying sex simply means sex (and frequency of sex) that is satisfying for *you*. There is no "right" number and there is no "right" way. Finally, consider asking your provider for a referral to a sex therapist.

Focus on Healing

Sexual difficulties are common; sleep issues are common. And *both* can grow even more difficult and complicated in midlife for a variety of reasons. But the good news is there are strategies to improve both our sleep *and* our sex.[8] Routinely practicing the following solutions for **bedroom hygiene** can help both issues *at the very same time*. How amazing is that?!?

1. **Establish that your bedroom (and your bed, specifically) is *only* used for two activities:** Sleep and sex. This means no TV. No work. No snacking. And no fighting.
2. **Create a regular sleep schedule.** Set an alarm for the same time every morning (maybe an hour or so later on weekends, if you prefer) and have a set bedtime. Make sure your schedule allows for seven to eight hours of time in your bed for rest/sleep.
3. **Eliminate brain-stimulating or anxiety-provoking behaviors before bed.** An hour before your scheduled bedtime, take a warm bath or read a calming book or ask your spouse for a shoulder massage. Be sure to put away your phone and switch off the news, and if you absolutely *must*

have some TV time on the couch to unwind, then put on a familiar show you've seen a hundred times before (I prefer *The Office* or *Schitt's Creek*). Whatever you choose, be sure to follow a similar routine night after night. Your brain will appreciate all the positive cues for sleep (and sex!).

4. **Exercise regularly to complete the stress cycle.** Daily exercise will work wonders on your sleep! But be sure to get your exercise at least two hours before heading to bed because the endorphins following exercise too close to bedtime can contribute to keeping you awake.

5. **Eliminate daytime naps.** You're tired, I know. But your brain thrives on routine, and sleeping during the day will only interrupt your set schedule and your body's circadian rhythm. It's super hard but super necessary. If you absolutely must close your eyes for a quick snooze, limit your nap time to twenty minutes or less.

6. **Stop caffeine intake after lunchtime.** This one is also extremely difficult to stick to, but it's essential for a good night of restful sleep.

7. **Allow for a change of venue.** If you wake during the night and can't get back to sleep, give yourself what feels like fifteen minutes to lie in bed. Don't check the clock or your phone, and if you still can't sleep, get up and go to a different room. Keep the lights low and do some quiet reading or turn on a show that typically puts you to sleep, and once you feel sleepy, head back to bed. Giving yourself permission to move to a new location helps alleviate any anxiety you may feel over not sleeping. Your brain will come to know you always have the option of simply changing the venue.

8. **Make time for intimacy.** Connect with your partner throughout the day. Let your hand brush across your

spouse's back or send a sexy text saying you're thinking of them and can't wait for later. Maybe schedule a date night with a *plan* for sex on the calendar if you need to so you can keep sex and connection in your relationship front and center in your mind.

9. **Share the following tips about *connection* with your spouse:**

- Instead of sleeping in or rushing off to work, roll over for a minute and kiss your wife. Like, reeeeaaaallly kiss her (this may work in your favor *right* on the spot).

- Catch her in the closet while she changes clothes and let your eyes linger, then tell her she's even more beautiful now than the day you first saw her.

- Send her a text from work to say, "I sure *love* doing life with you."

- When you get home (after you've read the room regarding any daily disasters and her openness to your touch), wrap your arms around her waist and lightly kiss the back of her neck while she's cooking at the stove, then ask about her day and really listen to her response.

- Work beside her on dinner dishes and bedtime, and once the kids are tucked into bed as she flops down on the couch exhausted from a long, hard day say, "I probably don't tell you often enough, but you're a really great mom."

- Take the initiative to foster deep passion as a couple throughout the day . . . and when you give the look on the way up to bed that says, *Hey, you wanna?*, I bet her look back will say, *I've been waiting ALL day for bedtime, and tonight it has nothing to do with sleep!*

10. **Keep an open mind.** Don't forget about date night and trying new things such as a vibrator device for extra stimulation to keep your relationship fresh and liven things up in the bedroom.

11. **Use a topical treatment.** Treat pain with intercourse due to vaginal dryness or other GSM with vaginal lubricants or moisturizers available over the counter. If that doesn't help, you may need to visit your doctor to get a prescription for a topical estrogen cream or other MHT if necessary.[9]

12. **Consider getting extra help.** A specialist in sleep medicine and/or a sex therapist may prove beneficial.

Please know, you're worth it. You really do deserve both connected and satisfying sex with your partner *and* regular restful sleep!

11

DIETARY AND "NATURAL" SUPPLEMENTS

Which Ones Do You Need?

Following my third grader's championship soccer game last year, the team met at a frozen yogurt shop to celebrate their loss. It was *so* hot, and the boys played *so* hard. Plus, frozen yogurt always sounds healthier than ice cream, doesn't it? Ice cream is full of sugar and fat and other "terrible" things that will begin to clog a person's arteries or cause diabetes, right? But yogurt? Surely that's a healthier alternative.

The yogurt place was a do-it-yourself kind of shop where you pick whatever flavor you like from giant machines and squeeze out a frozen yogurt snake that curls into your little paper bowl with pictures of cartoon fruits printed on the side. There were so many fun flavors to choose from like mango, banana, raspberry, chocolate, vanilla, strawberry, mint. My son chose vanilla.

"Vanilla goes with *any* topping, right, Mom?" Sure, buddy. Go ahead. You get whatever you want. Whatever sounds good to you. It's your day to celebrate.

Behind the frozen yogurt machines toward the back of the shop, we came upon a double row of very long counters lined with big canisters heaped over with every type of candy or topping imaginable. A veritable candy smorgasbord for children with Reese's, caramel, hot fudge, strawberry glaze, marshmallows, sprinkles, crushed Oreos, nuts, whipped cream, and maraschino cherries.

I watched my son's eyes widen and thought, *Oh this is so fun for him! He's having such a great time!* I felt like a good mom grabbing a little sweet treat at the frozen yogurt shop with my son and his teammates after their soccer game. Then I got distracted talking to the other mothers about school and our kids and how busy we are and David's mom's cute new sandals. *Where did she get those?* We laughed and talked and generally paid no attention to our children at the candy smorgasbord counter. And when my son reached the front of the line to pay for his yogurt creation, he turned and called to me, "Okay, Mom. I'm done. I'm ready."

My jaw dropped at what he plunked down on the scale.

His little bowl of "healthy" vanilla yogurt spilled over with *every single topping* available. M&M's and Reese's. Caramel and hot fudge. Marshmallows. Gummy worms. Sprinkles. Sour Patch Kids. Crushed Oreos. Twix. He must've added one little spoonful from every single heaping candy cannister. Then he plopped a dollop of whipped cream and one perfect round maraschino cherry on the top.

It cost $14.89.

We found a table next to the window with his teammates, where the boys laughed and talked and generally paid no attention to the parents, who eyed them warily as they threw back all that candy (which we felt sure would lead to diabetes, possibly by later that night). Then on the drive home, my son clutched at his stomach. And groaned. "I shoulda just had hot fudge."

It was a wonderful lesson in excess.

❋ ❋ ❋ ❋

I once treated a woman named Linda who downed "all natural" and "healthy" vitamins and herbal supplements like candy from that candy counter at the frozen yogurt shop.

Linda was fifty-one and postmenopausal. As a breast cancer survivor, she took great care of herself and had always been fairly health conscious. She was regimented about taking her daily prescription medications—a thyroid medication for hypothyroidism and a blood pressure medication that served two purposes: to keep her once-elevated blood pressure within the healthy range plus offer protection for her kidneys from any damaging effects of prediabetes. When we checked her labs every six months her cholesterol numbers were always at goal, and her blood sugar levels remained in the mildly elevated range consistent with prediabetes (which we'll talk more about in chapter 12) for which she chose dietary and lifestyle changes for treatment.

Linda scheduled healthcare maintenance exams on time and had her blood work done every six months and went to her follow-up mammogram appointments like clockwork. She ate healthily, for the most part. And, though she took a ten-minute walk over her lunch hour every single day, we both agreed she could be better about getting more rigorous exercise and prioritizing rest and sleep.

Linda struggled off and on with her mood and multiple midlife stressors, which included tying up loose ends following a very messy divorce. She had taken an SSRI for depression in the past but felt her mood was holding up okay despite the circumstances, and she was seeing a therapist regularly to help her through. She often made appointments with me in the clinic to discuss ongoing bowel symptoms consistent with **irritable bowel syndrome (IBS)**, a disorder which causes both recurrent abdominal pain related to bowel movements and changes in stool consistency that can involve constipation, diarrhea, or a mixed presentation of both.

Her initial blood work (which included a complete blood count and C-reactive protein level looking for inflammation) and colonoscopy were normal. Then during a follow-up appointment to discuss further normal blood work that included a blood panel to rule out celiac disease, Linda mentioned a ginseng supplement she was taking for its anti-inflammatory effects, hoping to improve her IBS symptoms. As we talked more, she mentioned a few other "natural" supplements she was taking for various reasons: turmeric, elderberry, garlic, cranberry, a probiotic . . .

I stopped her to ask, "Hey, Linda, do you happen to have a list of all the supplements you take?"

"Hmmm, no. I don't really keep a list. I just line the bottles up on my bathroom counter so I can remember to take them every morning."

"I see. Do you know roughly how many different supplements you're taking?"

"Oh, not really. I guess it's quite a few because I love Dr. Oz." She laughed. "He always gives the best suggestions for things I should take to stay healthy!"

I asked her to bring the bottles along with her to our next appointment together so we could document which supplements she was taking in addition to the prescription medications listed in her medical chart. When I saw her again a few weeks later, I was shocked to find over forty bottles of various "natural" vitamins and herbal supplements stacked two-high on the countertop next to her chair. We went through them one by one:

Glucosamine chondroitin

Turmeric

Elderberry

Vitamin C

Zinc

Vitamin B6 and B12 complex

Ashwagandha

Vitamin A

A daily supplement for "thyroid support"

Beta-carotene

Folic acid

Garlic

Green tea

A daily supplement for "memory support"

Cranberry

Ginseng

Echinacea

L-Lysine

CoQ-10

Three different probiotics

A fiber gummy

Omega-3 fatty acid

A daily supplement for "hair and nail health"

Magnesium

Calcium

Vitamin D

A daily multivitamin

It was a truly astonishing list. Many of the supplements on the list overlapped in their benefits—several claimed to be anti-inflammatory or heart healthy, many were for digestive health or immune function, several were for increased energy, joint health, or nerve function. And many turned out to be outright duplicates—the very same supplement being taken both individually *and* in either the multivitamin or her "thyroid support" combination supplement. Plus, many of these "all natural" herbal supplements cost more than $20–30 to fill every few months, depending on the size of the bottle and dosing recommendations. The bottles of pills spilling over the countertop in that little exam room likely added up to thousands of dollars per year!

It's important to remember here that "natural" supplements are pharmacologically active, meaning they can both positively and negatively impact our health. Supplements may provide the benefit we are looking for, but they may also cause side effects and drug interactions with other medications, foods, vitamins, or the other supplements we ingest. None of the individual supplements on Linda's list were known to be outright dangerous (though in some proprietary blends we're not exactly sure what's in there and sometimes safety testing is lacking), but I asked if she would be okay going through them together. When she agreed, I held up each bottle and asked a few questions:

> Why are you taking this?
>
> Do you know what benefit this supplement is supposed to bring?
>
> Have you noticed a difference since you started taking it?
>
> Is it helping you? Is it doing what it promises?
>
> Are there any harmful side effects from taking it?
>
> Does it overlap with any of the other supplements on this list?
>
> Does it interact with any of your prescription medications?
>
> Can you get what you need from this supplement through your diet instead?
>
> Have you researched negative long-term consequences from taking it?
>
> Do you really *need* it?

Digging Deeper into Supplements

Dietary supplements are sold to us as part of that $4.4 trillion "beauty and wellness" industry we talked about in chapter 1. They are branded as "wellness promoting," helping us achieve the world's health and beauty standard of thinness, anti-aging, optimal energy, and eternal youth from the inside out. We tend to believe supplements are superior to prescription medications produced by pharmaceutical companies because of the frequent use of buzz words in their elaborate marketing schemes like *natural,*

175

green, plant-based, organic, non-GMO[1] (though they don't always have the scientific support to make those claims). Plus, supplements are often emphasized by naturopaths, providers who sell that particular product, and other alternative-type healers. But, as with all medications and medical interventions, we need to cut through the noise and focus on whether each product is safe, effective, and indicated.

Let's start by reviewing the major issue with natural supplements we touched on in chapter 7, namely that the supplement industry is widely *unregulated*, and many of these "natural" products are missing the necessary safeguards for consumers. Supplements are not subject to the same federal regulations as prescription medications, which means they may not be uniform from bottle to bottle, may include contaminants, often come with a lack of safety testing, might be largely untested and unproven, and almost always come with exaggerated claims and very effective marketing based primarily on exploiting our pain points and fear. In fact, the only thing required of an "all natural," herbal, or dietary supplement before making its way to the shelf for sale is the following sentence after any claim about the product's general use:

> This statement has not been evaluated by the Food and Drug Administration. This product is not intended to diagnose, treat, cure, or prevent any disease.[2]

I'm sorry. I wish there were a slicker or more "holistic" sounding way. I wish I had a quick and easy answer. I wish I had a tidier truth to tell. But rather than popping back a lengthy list of herbal products or "natural" supplements that are "not intended to diagnose, treat, cure, or prevent any disease," please know that the very best way for most of us to get the nutrients we need every day is by eating a variety of healthy, nutrient-dense foods at every meal.

Though supplements may be useful or even necessary for those with an absorptive issue due to a medical illness such as celiac disease or for those who eat vegan or follow another special or restrictive diet to help fill in the gaps such diets may lack, in many cases supplements can actually *reduce* absorption of other nutrients from the diet and may cause adverse interactions with one another or with prescription medications. At the very least, taking a lengthy list of natural supplements produces very expensive urine because our bodies naturally pee any excess water-soluble vitamins right out.

Sometimes too much is simply too much. Right?

For all the reasons I've touched on here, Linda and I decided to do an experiment. She stopped taking her mixed grill of vitamins and herbal supplements and continued taking only her daily prescription medications, her omega-3 fatty acid supplement, and calcium with vitamin D. I encouraged her to focus on healthy eating and increase fiber in her diet along with plenty of water. And that was it.

She followed up in six weeks. And guess what? It didn't cure her IBS. Or her prediabetes. Or the situational anxiety she was experiencing off and on because of her recent messy divorce. But it did, however, improve the *frequency* of her IBS symptoms. Linda began having daily bowel movements that were mostly normal in consistency except for the occasional (less than once a month) flare of diarrhea symptoms that largely correlated with stressful events. And her abdomen remained mostly free of pain. Her symptoms (and definitely her savings account!) improved with *less*.

Focus on Healing

Now before you stop reading and hurl this book across the room, I want you to know I am not "anti" all vitamins or supplements or "anti" all alternative medicine treatments. I'm not. I simply want the supplements or alternative medicine treatments you are taking (and paying your hard-earned money for) to make sense. I want you to be well informed. I want you to refer to the questions I provided in chapter 2 about how to determine the validity and reliability of any "scientific" studies that tout a product's success. (Remember: sample size is important, third-party randomized, double-blinded, placebo-controlled testing is important, and replicability is important.) And I want you to be able to answer the same questions I posed to Linda, which basically boil down to

1. Is it safe?
2. Is it effective?
3. Is it indicated for *you*?

For each of the supplements you are currently taking, hold up the bottle and ask yourself:

- Why am I taking this?
- Is it helping?
- Are there any side effects or negative interactions with other medications I am taking?
- Could I get it through my diet instead?
- Do I really *need* it?

I encourage you to eliminate unnecessary dietary vitamins or supplements today. Also, be sure to let your medical providers know everything you do end up taking so they can be fully informed on your care and keep an updated list of both prescription medications and natural supplements in your medical record.

So, *which supplements do you* actually *need?*

Several vitamins/dietary supplements do meet the criteria of being safe, effective, and medically indicated, and for this reason, they are universally recommended from all medical communities based on sound medical research:

1. **Omega-3 fatty acids** lower triglycerides, reduce athero-sclerosis (thereby reducing heart attack and stroke), and decrease blood pressure. Foods with omega-3 fatty acids include ground flaxseed, walnuts, soybeans, enriched eggs, canola oil, fish, and other seafood. Prescription omega-3 fatty acid is called Omacor, and the typical dose is 1 g daily. Higher doses up to 4 g may treat elevated triglyc-erides and should always be monitored under the care of your physician. Side effects of omega-3 fatty acids may include nausea, diarrhea, heartburn, and bad breath.[3]

2. **Calcium** is important for bone health, and for those who can't get enough through their diet, a supplement is rec-ommended. The total daily requirement for women is 1,000 to 1,200 mg. Foods with calcium include dairy prod-ucts, fortified soy or almond milk, tofu, chia seeds, kale, figs, and sardines. A calcium supplement combined with vitamin D is recommended since vitamin D helps with absorption of calcium. A side effect of taking calcium may include kidney stones.[4]

3. **Vitamin D** helps the body absorb calcium, improves muscle health, and promotes a healthy immune system. The recommended daily intake for vitamin D from a com-bination of both dietary intake and supplementation is 800 to 1,000 IU a day. Vitamin D3 is made in the skin from exposure to ultraviolet B rays from the sun. Vitamin D3 is also found in liver, butter, eggs, and fatty fish. Many other foods are now fortified with vitamin D2. Both vitamin D2 and D3 are converted to calcitriol, which is the usable form in the body. In general, vitamin D supplementa-tion within the recommended range does not cause side effects.[5]

4. **Fiber** is essential for optimal health and nutrition. Dietary fiber works to provide bulk and give a feeling of fullness

179

after a meal. It increases the volume of stool to reduce constipation. It levels out the blood sugar spike that occurs after eating. And it reduces total cholesterol. Because of all these amazing effects, a high-fiber diet lowers the rates of colon cancer, diabetes, and cardiovascular diseases like heart attacks and stroke. Women should aim for 25 g of dietary fiber per day. Dietary fiber is found in whole grains, certain fruits and vegetables, and legumes. Side effects of fiber may include bloating and gas.[6]

I know. We want *the answer*, and mostly we'd like that answer to be relatively easy. We want to take good care of our bodies, but eating well and exercising regularly and getting enough rest and remembering to floss and hauling our bodies to all those health-care maintenance exams just seems . . . HARD. *I mean, isn't there a supplement or two I can take? An herb I can steep in my tea? Maybe the powdered stem cells of an orchid I can add to my pre-workout drink instead?* We long for the quick fix (with bonus points if that fix appears to be "all natural"). But the truth is, if it sounds too good to be true, then it really is too good to be true.

So, can we agree? If a supplement or medical intervention or alternative treatment is safe, effective, and indicated with sound medical science to back it, then it's probably a good idea. But if not, then we're simply better off without it. All the money we'll save by eliminating unnecessary herbal and "natural" products will simply be the cherry on top!

12

PREVENTIVE CARE
FOR WOMEN IN MIDLIFE

The thing about life is often it does not behave the way we wish it would. Instead, just when we're managing to limp along rather nicely, getting to work on time, and somehow serving up a hot dinner around the table a few nights a week or occasionally having sweet conversations with our surly teenager over a plate of ten p.m. nachos, WHAM! A breast lump appears.

Plus, life almost *never* plays the fairness game. Like, if you've already been through a terrible bout of cancer of say, the stomach, with a tumor for which you will chronically be on immunotherapy—an awful medication that drains your energy and makes you gain weight despite frequent nausea and may even cause your hair to thin—life never decides that you've had your fair share of bad luck or hard times and perhaps for this next thing you should be spared. Nope. The breast lump you found could still be cancer.

This is why the medical community proposes preventive care with regular healthcare maintenance exams and screening tests and annual blood work. Because sometimes finding something *early* takes the sting away, and instead of being jerked cleanly off your feet, you'll be able to do something about it before the total knock-out punch. And this is why, occasionally, we entice you to schedule your mammogram by offering a bunch of yummy snacks with a pair of free socks as a bonus.

That's how it went for my friend Jessica. She made the appointment to get her screening mammogram because of the promise of free socks. She didn't have any breast cancer in the family. She hadn't noticed any new lumps or anything abnormal. Plus, her mammogram had been completely normal two years before. Not to mention she was still taking immunotherapy for a gastrointestinal stromal tumor (GIST) of the stomach that was diagnosed a few years prior. Another primary cancer would not be fair for her, right?

Jess wanted the free socks. And what they found was a ductal carcinoma in situ of her breast which, after surgical excision with a lumpectomy and a few rounds of radiation, required no further treatment other than frequent monitoring. If she had waited until symptoms appeared—a lump or mass or an itching sensation around her nipple or noticeable dimpling of the skin—her breast cancer would've progressed enough to require much more invasive treatment like a mastectomy, chemotherapy, more extensive radiation, and/or ongoing oral medications. Jess's story brings some real-world credibility to the importance of preventive health care. And her unique situation could happen to any one of us. So, let's talk more about preventive health care and the importance of regular checkups and screening exams.

Digging Deeper into Prevention

The goal of preventive care is ultimately to prevent disease, disability, and death as well as improve overall well-being. Prevention can be broken down into three types:[1]

In **primary prevention**, the goal is to intervene before any illnesses occur. Examples of primary prevention include vaccinations, a healthy diet, and not smoking or using illicit substances. The focus of primary prevention is to prevent disease.

In **secondary prevention**, the goal is to discover disease in an early stage and intervene before the full range of symptoms develops. An example of secondary prevention is treating high cholesterol or high blood pressure before obvious heart disease. The focus of secondary prevention is early diagnosis and prompt treatment.

In **tertiary prevention**, the goal is to decrease the long-term effects of the disease after a diagnosis has been made. An example of tertiary prevention is treating those with type 2 diabetes with an ace-inhibitor medication to protect against kidney damage. The focus of tertiary prevention is slowing or stopping disease progression.

Prevention is an important aspect of good health and essential healing; however, it is simply impossible to screen for every possible medical condition. So how does the medical community decide which illnesses to screen for? There are three main points to consider:

- The condition being screened for must be an important, common, and relatively universal health problem.
- The condition must have an early stage in which treatment makes a difference in long-term outcomes—which means screening for, finding, and beginning treatment early makes a difference in the overall **morbidity** (a term for *suffering* due to illness) and **mortality** (a term for *death* due to illness) of that condition.
- The screening test for the condition must be accurate, easy to administer, widely available, relatively comfortable, and relatively inexpensive with a high degree of **sensitivity**, meaning cases of disease will not be missed.

In general, regular healthcare maintenance visits with your healthcare provider will evaluate your personal risk factors for illness, discuss any new symptoms you are experiencing, review your current lifestyle practices and suggest healthy changes toward healing, highlight the importance of mental health, and focus on preventive care specific to *you*. For women younger than fifty without underlying chronic medical illness, preventive health visits are recommended every three years. After age fifty, these visits are recommended annually.

Let's continue now by highlighting within each organ system the preventive examinations, screening tests, and lifestyle modifications essential to women for health and healing during midlife. Screening tests and preventive care specific to transgender individuals with past or current hormone use can be found in appendix 4.

Heart Health

Cardiovascular disease is the leading cause of death for all women in the United States and is responsible for one in every five female deaths. This is yet another area where health disparities persist, and Black women are at increased risk of both morbidity and mortality from cardiovascular disease. Nearly half of Black women over the age of twenty years already have evidence of heart disease. Preventive health care for the heart focuses on the **modifiable risk factors** for cardiovascular disease, which means if we can intervene and make positive changes in these areas, then the risk for cardiovascular death decreases substantially.

Modifiable risk factors we regularly assess and treat to prevent cardiovascular disease[2]

- Screen for **hypertension** (or high blood pressure) every year.
  - A normal blood pressure reading is <130/80.
  - 135/85 is consistent with elevated blood pressure.
  - And 140/90 on two separate occasions means a diagnosis of hypertension can be made and should be treated either with medication or lifestyle changes (likely both).

- Check total cholesterol levels for **hyperlipidemia** (or high cholesterol) at least every five years beginning at age 35 for women who have other risk factors or age 45 for women without underlying risks until age 65.
  - Instead of looking at the total cholesterol, we need to focus on the individual parts that make up that total. I've lost count of how many times a friend has called with concerns about a high cholesterol result, wondering if she will have to eat dry salads and chicken breast from here on out. But when we look together at the breakdown of her cholesterol numbers, it turns out that her numbers aren't high, they are *ideal*. And her total cholesterol only appears high due to a very high HDL.
  - Optimal cholesterol results look like this:
    - Total cholesterol 125–200 mg/dL
    - LDL (or "bad" cholesterol) <100 mg/dL (generally the lower the better)
    - HDL (or "good" cholesterol) >40 mg/dL (generally the higher the better)
    - Triglycerides <150 mg/dL
- Assess for **type 2 diabetes** every year beginning at age 35 until age 75 using one of the following screening tests:
  - A fasting blood glucose level
    - A normal fasting blood glucose level is <100.
    - A fasting glucose level 100–125 is consistent with **pre-diabetes** (and about 10% of people with prediabetes will become diabetic within a year without any lifestyle modifications or medication).
    - A fasting glucose level >126 on two occasions is diagnostic for type 2 diabetes.
  - A hemoglobin A1C level
    - A normal HgA1C is <5.7%.

How you can prevent cardiovascular disease

- Stop smoking.
- Get regular aerobic exercise.
  - Aim for 150 minutes of moderate-intensity or 75 minutes of vigorous-intensity aerobic exercise every week alongside at least two days of muscle strengthening and daily stretching/balance training.
- Eat a diet with plenty of fruits and vegetables, lean protein, healthy fats, and whole grains and limit saturated fats, sugar, and highly processed foods like fast food.
- Limit alcohol use.
- Be aware of heart symptoms in women: chest fullness rather than pain, nausea, heartburn, tiredness, shortness of breath, or feeling lightheaded.

Breast Health

Breast cancer is the leading non-skin cause of cancer in women and the second deadliest cancer for women worldwide. Black women are at increased risk. When early detection and up-to-date treatments are available, the five-year survival rate for early breast cancer (that has not yet spread to lymph nodes or other organs) exceeds 80%. Therefore, the goal of breast cancer screening is to detect breast cancer at an early stage.[3]

How we screen for breast cancer[4]

- Digital mammography is the standard breast cancer screening tool. A mammogram is an X-ray of the breast, and results are available within a matter of days. About one in ten women who have a mammogram will need further imaging either with a repeat mammogram, MRI, or ultrasound.

- A clinical breast exam by a trained physician may provide only a modest improvement in detection, so these exams are no longer routinely recommended as part of breast cancer screening. An in-office breast exam *is* helpful if you noticed a lump at home that needs to be evaluated.

- Regular self-breast examinations have failed to display a benefit and may actually cause unnecessary anxiety, cost, and pain from unneeded imaging and/or breast biopsies. These exams are no longer routinely recommended as part of breast cancer screening.

When to screen for breast cancer

- Your healthcare provider will begin recommending regular mammograms every one to two years starting at the age of 40, 45, or 50. The age to start screening depends on your risk of developing breast cancer, which depends on genetics (like whether you carry the BRCA 1 or BRCA 2 gene or have a family history with multiple close relatives with breast cancer) and other risk factors such as increasing age, your reproductive/menstrual history, having dense breasts, alcohol or tobacco use, and obesity.[5]

- In general, women should continue regular screening mammograms for as long as their life expectancy is at least ten more years.

Bone Health

With age, our bones become less dense, which means our bones become thinner, more fragile, and prone to fractures following minor injuries. The fancy word for this thinning of bone is **osteoporosis**. Up to 20% of women over the age of 50 years will have evidence of osteoporosis on bone density tests. This number increases after menopause to up to 70% of women by age 85. Early treatment for osteoporosis can reduce the risk for fracture, thus reducing the decreased mobility and decreased quality of life that can result from a hip fracture.[6]

How we screen for osteoporosis

- Regular bone density testing with **duel-energy X-ray ab-sorptiometry (DEXA)** scanning evaluates the level of bone thinning and can provide an estimate of fracture risk. Testing should be repeated every two to ten years depending on the initial results and your underlying risk factors.[7]

When to screen for osteoporosis

- All women older than 65 years of age should have a bone density test at least once. Those with risk factors for osteoporosis—such as previously breaking a bone as an adult, a history of hip fracture, taking oral steroids regularly, having low body weight, tobacco or alcohol use, or having rheumatoid arthritis or other secondary causes for osteoporosis—will need even earlier bone density testing.[8]

How you can prevent fractures related to decreased bone density

- Get an adequate amount of calcium (1200 mg daily) and vitamin D (800 IU daily) through dietary intake and supplements if necessary.
- Exercise regularly with weight-bearing exercises like walking or running, strength training with weights or bands, and balance/flexibility training using stretching exercises or yoga.
- Stop smoking.
- Limit alcohol use.
- Take osteoporosis medications if bone density tests reveal low bone density.

Bowel Health

Colon and rectal cancer (which we squish together and call **colorectal cancer**) is common and deadly. Colorectal cancer is the second most common cancer diagnosed in women, and—yep, you guessed it—Black women are at increased risk. Finding cancer early by detecting and removing polyps helps prevent widespread cancer and improves long-term outcomes. So, just like for breast cancer, the goal of colorectal cancer screening is to detect colorectal cancer at an early stage.[9]

Options we use to screen for colorectal cancer[10]

- Colonoscopy is the standard colorectal cancer screening tool because it allows for direct visualization inside the entire colon. Typically, the prep prior to getting a colonoscopy is the worst part because the colon must be cleaned out using a medication that causes very watery diarrhea. During the colonoscopy procedure, medication is given for comfort, and most people don't remember anything about having the exam. If polyps are found during the exam, they can be removed on the spot. In general, a colonoscopy is required every ten years.

- Because colorectal cancer tends to cause microscopic bleeding into the stool that we can't see, stool testing for blood every year is another way to test for colorectal cancer. If this stool test comes back positive, then a colonoscopy is required.

- Sigmoidoscopy is similar to colonoscopy except it evaluates only the last part of the colon and rectum. Prior to this test, an enema is used to clean out the colon, and during the procedure, medications for relaxation or comfort are not required. Sigmoidoscopy should be repeated every five to ten years. And if polyps or other abnormalities are found, then a full colonoscopy is required.

When to screen for colorectal cancer

- Your healthcare provider will likely begin recommending colorectal cancer screening at age 45.[11] Those with increased risk—such as women with a strong family history of colon cancer or those with a personal history of Crohn's disease or ulcerative colitis, which are two inflammatory conditions of the bowel—will need screening at a younger age.

- In general, most people can stop colon cancer screening at age 75 or, at the latest, 85.

Gynecologic Health

The organs of the female reproductive system—the uterus, ovaries, fallopian tubes, cervix, and external genitalia—continue to require medical attention and monitoring after the childbearing years have passed whether or not you have had children. During healthcare maintenance visits, your doctor will review your menstrual cycle and menstrual history and assess any risks you have for sexually transmitted infections (STI), the need for contraception (because remember, until menopause you can still get pregnant), any urinary complaints, and your personal risk factors for cancers of the reproductive system, including cervical cancer.

The number one cause of cervical cancer is infection with human papilloma virus (HPV), which can be transmitted through *any kind* of sexual contact. At least 80% of women will be exposed to HPV in their lifetime, and for most, the immune system does a great job of clearing the virus without long-term consequences. In some cases, however, certain strains of HPV can lead to precancerous and cancerous lesions of the cervix that are highly treatable in the early stages of disease.[12] So, once again, early detection is key.

Options we use to screen for cervical cancer[13]

- A Papanicolaou (pap) test, also called a "pap smear," collects a small sample of cells by gently scraping the cervix during a pelvic exam and should generally be repeated every three years.
- Co-testing, which is a combination of HPV testing along with a pap smear, is another way to screen by collecting a sample of cells from the cervix *and* using a swab to test for HPV infection and should generally be repeated every five years.

When to screen for cervical cancer[14]

- Age 21–29 = begin screening with a pap smear every three years
- Age 30–65 = continue screening with a pap smear every three years *or* with either co-testing or HPV testing every five years
- Age 65+ = no further screening is necessary *if* all previous pap smears have been normal OR there have been either three normal pap smears or two normal co-tests over the past ten years with the most recent test within the past five years
- Women who have had a total hysterectomy (which includes removal of the cervix) do not need to be screened for cervical cancer.

How you can prevent HPV infection

- The greatest protection from HPV infection is to be vaccinated *before* sexual activity begins. For this reason, routine HPV vaccination is recommended for all children ages 11 to 12 when only two doses are needed. "Catch up" vaccination is recommended for all people up to 26 years of age who have not yet been vaccinated with three doses.[15]

- The vaccine is approved for use through the age of 45 for those who have not been vaccinated. Indications for vaccination in this age group vary by the individual.

In average-risk women, there is no evidence to support regular screening for other gynecologic cancers since routine testing does *not* improve overall morbidity or mortality. Furthermore, screening tests for these types of cancer can be associated with a high number of false positive tests, leading to invasive testing or unnecessary procedures and surgeries, which can be both painful and costly. Any testing of your uterus, ovaries, or other reproductive organs must be based on your underlying risk factors and whether you develop any abnormal symptoms, which should be routinely discussed at a yearly healthcare maintenance exam with your provider.

Skin, Eye, and Dental Health

All adults with a high risk for **melanoma**, which is an aggressive form of skin cancer, should have a regular full-body skin exam every year. Risks for melanoma include a history of skin cancer, a family history of melanoma, white race, fair skin with a propensity for sunburn, a total number of moles greater than fifty, or immune suppression due to illness or medication.

Also, eye examinations to assess vision, determine eye pressures, and evaluate the optic nerve are recommended annually as well as dental visits every six months.[16]

Lung Health

All adults between the ages of 50 to 80 years with a twenty pack-year history of smoking who currently smoke or who quit smoking within the last fifteen years should have yearly lung cancer screening with a low-dose CT scan.[17] A **pack-year** is calculated by multiplying the number of packs of cigarettes smoked per day by the number of years smoked.

Immunizations

It's been proven again and again that immunizations are an effective way to prevent disease; however, the timing and dosing recommendations for a particular immunization may change. In general, an updated Covid-19 vaccine and a flu shot is recommended every year. Others to consider with increasing age and discuss with your provider include the shingles (zoster) vaccine and the pneumonia (pneumococcal) vaccine. The Centers for Disease Control and Prevention (CDC) puts out updated recommendations every year based on new and emerging evidence and ongoing research. You'll find the most recent chart on the next page.[18]

Mental Health

Since it is estimated that less than 50% of depression cases are identified without the use of a screening tool, *and* treatment for major depression is more effective when started early in the course of illness, regular screening for depression using the PHQ-2 questionnaire, which we discussed in chapter 9, is recommended for all adults at each healthcare maintenance exam. If the PHQ-2 questionnaire screens positive, the PHQ-9 can more accurately evaluate depressive symptoms and assign a level of severity of mild, moderate, or severe. Again, the PHQ-9 can be found in appendix 3.

❋ ❋ ❋ ❋

Preventive care is important for our ongoing health and healing. I was reminded of that in a deeply personal way when I had dinner with my friend Jessica recently. We laughed and talked and enjoyed spending time together. She told me about her promotion at work, where she is now the nurse manager of her hospital's med-surg

Recommended Adult Immunization Schedule by Age Group

Vaccine	19-26 years	27-49 years	50-64 years	≥65 years
Covid-19*	1 or more doses of updated (2023-2024 Formula) vaccine (See Notes)			
Influenza inactivated (IIV4) or Influenza recombinant (RIV4)	1 dose annually			
Influenza live, attenuated (LAIV4)	1 dose annually			
Tetanus, diphtheria, pertussis (Tdap or Td)	1 dose Tdap each pregnancy; 1 dose Td/Tdap for wound management (see notes)			
	1 dose Tdap, then Td or Tdap booster every 10 years			
Measles, mumps, rubella (MMR)	1 or 2 doses depending on indication (if born in 1957 or later)			For healthcare professional (see notes)
Varicella (VAR)	2 doses (if born in 1980 or later)		2 doses	
Zoster recombinant (RZV)	2 doses for immunocompromising conditions (see notes)			2 doses
Human papillomavirus (HPV)	2 or 3 doses depending on age at initial vaccination or condition	27 through 45 years		
Pneumococcal (PCV15, PCV20, PPSV23)	See notes			See notes
				See notes
Hepatitis A (HepA)	2, 3, or 4 doses depending on vaccine			
Hepatitis B (HepB)	2, 3, or 4 doses depending on vaccine or condition			
Meningococcal A, C, W, Y (MenACWY)	1 or 2 doses depending on indication, see notes for booster recommendations			
Meningococcal B (MenB)	19 through 23 years	2 or 3 doses depending on vaccine and indication, see notes for booster recommendations		
Haemophilus influenzae type b (Hib)	1 or 3 doses depending on indication			
Mpox				

Legend:

- Recommended vaccination for adults who meet age requirement, lack documentation of vaccination or lack evidence of immunity
- Recommended vaccination for adults with an additional risk factor or another indication
- Recommended vaccination abased on shared clinical descision-making
- No recommendations/Not applicable

floor *and* the ortho-spine wing. We swapped a few stories about our growing teenagers and howled with laughter at the ridiculousness of being a mom to these hilarious and fun older kids.

She was so beautiful and full of life sitting across from me at the table. She *is* so beautiful and intelligent and loving and loyal and sarcastic and real and fun. And I am truly grateful for the advances of modern medicine—both the preventive measures and treatment modalities—that have kept her here. She is truly a gift to the world.

Be sure to see *your* doctor regularly. Stay up to date on your regular healthcare maintenance needs and screening exams. Make it a top priority to take very good care of YOU—because *you* are a gift to the world, too. And hey, you might even get a pair of free socks!

13

SHAME-BASED "HEALTH" PRACTICES VS. LOVE-BASED HEALING

A Look at Trauma

Unspeakable and tortuous things can happen in life, and it changes us. Trauma *changes* us.

Sometimes trauma changes us, and we can survive it. We can reach beyond it to find something true and beautiful that helps us carry on. Move forward and find peace alongside the pain. Maybe even discover a little contentment and joy along the way. But sometimes trauma is so devastating that it changes us in a way we believe we can't escape. There is no peace, no love, no help, no comfort, and no healing. Instead, we feel desperate and alone. The unbearable trauma sets us on a path toward more pain and more hurt and even more trauma. Toward drugs and alcohol and sex and jail and more loss and shame and other traumatized people who will only exploit our unspeakable pain.

Years ago at the end of my residency, I spent two months working for a rural hospital as part of my training. I treated patients in the clinic during the day and worked in the tiny, four-bed emergency department overnight. On top of that, my duties included providing obstetrical care for pregnant inmates at the women's correctional facility in the area. Over the course of my eight weeks at that hospital, four brand-new babies were born to women from the correctional facility.

The women presented in labor to the hospital sweaty and cursing, tattooed and panting through pursed lips while wearing khaki-colored maternity jumpsuits and handcuffs. Many of them looked at me skeptically like, *Really? This girl is going to deliver my baby?* An armed guard stood just outside the door while I used the doppler to listen for fetal heart tones, checked for a dilated cervix, performed the necessary admission testing and an ultrasound, reviewed charts, wrote orders, and admitted the women to the hospital to assist with their active labor.

Most of them had wretched stories. Shocking, ghastly, horrible stories filled with physical abuse and drug use and felony charges, with previous incarcerations and abusive boyfriends and restraining orders, with growing-up years spent in and out of foster care, plus all manner of terrible, unspeakable tragedies endured throughout childhood. I cannot imagine the trauma these laboring women were carrying as they now had to birth a baby at the hands of a young, seemingly naïve white woman while an armed guard stood outside the door waiting to return them to jail, where they would have monitored visits with their newborns.

I was not technically qualified to deliver their babies independently, but I had plenty of experience in the delivery room and was confident in my abilities. And though I always called the attending physician upon each woman's admission to the hospital, often the doctor overseeing my work casually arrived only as I was finishing up the delivery note. I was on my own, but I wasn't afraid. It seemed to me that many of these women felt like they were alone. And though the women were skeptical of my presence, I felt honored to be beside them. To help them. To hold all the pain and sadness and devastation of their previous traumas while also bearing witness to the beauty of new life and their obvious motherly love.

One night a particularly gruff-looking woman who had been surly and distant on admission, barely acknowledging my existence and giving terse, one-word replies to my questions, screamed with abandon throughout the delivery as if screaming at the desperation of her entire situation. Of her entire life. When I plopped her pink, squalling baby boy upon her chest—exclaiming, "It's a boy!"—I noticed her whole face changed.

She looked up at me now with desperate eyes, childlike and pleading, "Is he okay? Is it all right? Doctor . . . did I do all right?"

It seemed like she was asking, *Am I lovable?*

"He's beautiful" was my reply. "He's *perfect*. You did *so* good. You are amazing."

Her eyes filled with tears at my response. Then she gazed adoringly upon her perfect new baby with the same kind of love I felt instantly for my first child—a mother's love—full of hope and promise and new beginnings. And my own child, my next baby boy already six months along, kicked and somersaulted inside me.

I wanted to tell her to let that animalistic, motherly love change her. Let it open her up. Let it teach her to reach for healing and grace, for something *beyond* her past trauma. I wanted to tell her to turn all that good and pure and primal love inward. Toward herself. Toward the little girl who was abused and hurt and cast aside and left alone so that instead of more pain and trauma and jail time, she could live the life that was *hers*. But I couldn't find the right words.

"Look at that," I said instead as her newborn snuggled into her chest. "He knows his momma."

She smiled back at me. For that moment, all the gruffness that had been hiding her pain was gone. And I will never forget her face. Trauma changes us, it's true. But *love* can change us, too.

❊ ❊ ❊

A decade or so later, I met Krystal. At the time, I worked as a "PRN" (or *pro re nata*) provider, which meant I worked a few days every month "as needed," moving from clinic to clinic around the Salt Lake City area filling in for providers who were sick or taking a much-needed vacation. My husband was years into recovery from his drug and alcohol use, and I'd had my fifth and final child earlier that summer. Since I worked in over twenty clinics in the area, every patient I treated was a new patient to me. And on one of those days, Krystal arrived.

Krystal was a *beautiful* human. She was loud and sarcastic and funny—a bright and boisterous ray of sunshine with big, wild red hair and giant black-gauge earrings, a smattering of freckles on the pale skin of her nose, and scads of colorful tattoos running up and down her arms. Krystal had the kind of reckless and wonderfully full laugh that made me wish she would simply keep laughing, and after two minutes in the exam room with Krystal's big personality, I was sure everywhere this beautiful human went, her contagious laugh and enormous warmth drew people in and made them feel at home. I felt certain that every day in a million ways, Krystal made people smile.

Krystal's appointment was a follow-up visit on her medication for anxiety and depression. I had already reviewed the previous office notes before heading into the exam room and knew she'd been taking Wellbutrin for six months without complications. So, we began by discussing the symptoms that made her come into the doctor's office in the first place and whether the medication was helping.

Krystal told me she restarted depression medication after moving into her apartment alone. She'd left her partner months before and still wasn't used to the quiet and loneliness of living alone. Plus, she wasn't currently speaking to her mother, who'd been an inconsistent presence in her life—on and off drugs, in and out of rehab, occasionally violent and abusive, often incarcerated, forever dating various mysterious and sometimes dangerous men, and generally leaving Krystal to fend for herself as a child. Krystal was working through those old childhood hurts and had done well on similar medication for depression symptoms in the past.

Krystal worked for an evening caregiver respite program providing care for elderly individuals still living at home or those with various disabilities. The pay was awful, and the work was demanding. Her working hours consisted of helping with meals and cleaning up around the house and changing adult-sized diapers until the family or caregivers could return, which was all quite messy and physically hard and emotionally demanding. Five days a week the shift ended at 9:30 p.m., but then to make ends meet, she worked twelve-hour shifts at a gas station on the weekends. Those two jobs brought in just enough money to cover rent for a one-bedroom apartment and utilities and the car payment for her used car.

She had been seeing a therapist regularly for a while but skipped her weekly appointments for the last few months. And as she told me about her job and her mother and her life, her voice sort of trailed away, "I'm fine, really." She looked up at me and smiled. "The medication . . . helps. And I just love my patients. My job and spending time with all those beautiful people who *need* me is how I keep going."

I almost turned toward the computer then and clicked a few buttons to send her medication order off to the pharmacy where it could be refilled. I almost concluded our visit and recommended she follow up in a few months with her regular provider. I almost stood up and left the room. But there was something about the way her voice trailed away that made me stay.

I didn't say anything. I didn't ask any more questions. I didn't move on to another topic. I just sat there. Waiting. Smiling gently. Leaning in a little and looking Krystal straight in her beautifully bright, green-hazel eyes.

I've learned there is a lot of power in the wait. There's just something about a good long pause that makes a person's mind begin searching, *Isn't she going to say anything? Wait, was there a question? Why is she just sitting there looking at me? Am I supposed to keep talking? Could I really just . . . keep talking?* Sometimes I wait long enough to make us both feel the slightest bit uncomfortable. But then, so often, it works. And my patient—or whoever I'm talking to—just keeps talking.

"Hey, Dr. Albertson? Can I tell you something?"

Krystal hesitated. And her eyes fell. Her once boisterous voice changed from contagious and full of light to quiet and tinged with a bit of fear and shame.

"I, uh, I can't really believe I'm telling you this. *I never told anybody about this.* But can I tell you what I do after work sometimes?" She looked down at her hands, fidgeting in her seat.

"Of course," I said, leaning a little farther forward on my doctor's stool.

"Well. Um. Sometimes after work, I stop off at the store and buy a case of beer. A whole case, you know?" She looked up briefly. "Then, um, when I get home, I go to my bedroom. And I pull this chair over to my closet, 'cause there's this big mirror on the outside," she explained, motioning with her hands. "Then I just kinda . . . sit there."

She paused again, twisting nervously at the rings on her fingers, staring distantly out the window at the trees rustling in the breeze outside while I waited.

"And I. Uh. I watch myself drink it in the mirror. Sometimes I drink a whooooole case. Myself. And most times, about halfway through it, I. Um. I. Start yellin' at the *ugly freak* I see looking back!"

She stopped then. Surprised. She looked back at me, obviously shocked by her own words. By the truth. Then fear and anger flickered in her eyes until suddenly her heart flooded open, and her unbearable pain spilled out in one big, long run-on sentence as tears dribbled down her cheeks and splashed into her mouth and across the tattoos decorating her neck.

"I *scream* at her and I curse at her and I tell her she's fat and stupid and worthless and I tell her I know exactly why everyone just leaves and I tell her how much I hate her. I HATE HER! Because . . . I just . . . I . . . *hate* her."

I didn't say a word as she continued, urgently; as if now that she started, she just *had* to keep talking. Had to get it all out. I reached my hand out to hers, squeezing firmly and trying to press in my love.

Her eyes were pleading now with mine. "And then, sometimes. I, uh. I break one of the tabs offa the cans? And I. Um. I. I start . . . cutting. You know? Twisting the sharp part into my arms or legs. It just feels good to dig it in there. It hurts; but it feels kinda good, too. You know? Like a . . . a . . . a release or something."

I looked down as she flipped her arm over to expose the small scars lining the edges of her forearm while I held tightly to her other hand, hoping to absorb some of her terrible pain.

"Do you think that means I'm crazy?" she pleaded.

I wanted to pull her onto my lap. I wanted to hold her and rock her and pat her gently on the back while humming *You Are My Sunshine* like I did with my little ones at home. I knew I couldn't, but I wanted to invite her into my car and drive her home and pull up a seat at the table with the rest of my family. I wanted to erase the memories of her childhood hurts. I wanted to fix the unbearable pain she carries through her days. I wanted to heal this beautiful woman's broken heart. I wanted more than anything in the whole world to take away the sadness in her eyes. I wanted her to know she is loved. *Loved, loved, loved.*

But it was only a thirty-minute office visit. And I was only working "as needed." And none of those things would be part of an appropriate doctor-patient relationship. And unfortunately, I deeply understand that sometimes it takes a whole lifetime to even begin to mend and heal from a broken past.

So, instead, I took both of her hands into mine. Then I stared into her wild green-hazel eyes overflowing with pain and fear and sadness and loss, and I said with the most sincere and loving voice I could muster, "No. Do you hear me? Krystal? No. I absolutely do not think you're crazy. I think you are hurt, and I think you need help, and I think this is what trauma does, and I am not going to leave you alone in it. Okay? I want you to stay. Stay, Krystal. Okay? Your patients. The whole world. We *all* need you. Here. You are wanted. You are so very loved. And I want you to stay."

I hugged her, then, and she clung to me tightly as I prayed silently with her in my arms. I held her. And I prayed that she would reach—*beyond the pain*—until she found something true and beautiful to help her carry on.

"Okay," she whispered into my shoulder. "I'll stay."

Digging Deeper into Trauma

Trauma happens when we are left to suffer alone after something horrible happens to us. Nearly all of us carry some type of pain from the past—physical, sexual, or emotional abuse; the devastating loss of a loved one; a terrible, messy divorce (perhaps our parents' divorce when we were children, or later, our own shocking divorce when something like infidelity knocks us flat); a disfiguring accident; or the silent, searing pain of some other terrible, unspeakable hurt. But the trauma only settles into our souls when we somehow believe we are alone in it. And it changes us. Gabor Maté explains trauma in his compelling book, *The Myth of Normal*:

> "Trauma" is an inner injury, a lasting rupture or split within the self due to difficult or hurtful events. By this definition, trauma is primarily what happens within someone as a result of the difficult or hurtful events that befall them; it is not the events themselves. "Trauma is not what happens *to* you but what happens *inside* you" is how I formulate it.[1]

Remember the results of the ACE study we discussed in chapter 3? Trauma *changes* us, and when we are left alone with our pain, it leaves a lasting wound on our bodies and souls.

I know because my father's father touched and fondled and groped me when I was a child. With my grandma napping in the next room, my grandfather entered my room to "play," and before I knew what was happening, he had grabbed me around the waist and pressed his bulging midsection into my back and pulled me backwards onto the bed—my little white daybed with the teddy bear comforter.

I was eight.

In that moment, a horrible feeling settled in my stomach that was eerily familiar to me. This had happened to me before. I had been sexually abused for years when I was four and five and six by a different relative at family reunions and Christmas get-togethers and Sunday night dinners. It was confusing to me at the time because I understood this other relative was a kid, just like me. Yet he was so big. His tongue felt enormous in my mouth. It hurt when he touched me and poked at me and prodded between my legs. And it seemed so strange when he wedged himself between my thighs and began pumping himself up and down, huffing above me. Generally, when the abuse happened, I floated away somewhere outside of my body until it was over. Until he was done. I wasn't there. Not really. But all of it left a particularly horrible feeling in my stomach. I didn't know how to make any of it stop. I didn't know how to tell anybody. And mostly, I just didn't want to hurt anyone with the truth.

I thought I'd left it all safely behind when we moved to another town, but then a few years later . . . there it was. My grandfather came to stay, and on my little white daybed with the teddy bear comforter when he touched and fondled and groped, that particular horrible feeling in my stomach returned. Again.

I had so many questions: Why did this keep happening to me? Why hadn't anyone been able to stop it? Why hadn't *I* been able to stop it? Why had I frozen? Why didn't I say something? And why . . . me?

But I didn't tell anyone about my abuse for decades, hoping my silence about it would make the truth disappear. *It wasn't that big a deal,* I told myself. *I never really said no to that other relative. I just never said anything at all. I simply froze. I should've said something,* I reasoned. *Plus, I wasn't wearing pants that first time it happened with my grandfather, so it must've been my fault. Why was I walking around the house in a T-shirt and underwear? Plus, it could have been worse. I was fine! I could control this. No one would ever have to know.*

Somehow, I became an adult when I was four or five or six years old lying on a creaky old cot in a cabin at a family reunion while that teenage relative did whatever he pleased with my naked little body. I kept myself safe by floating somewhere above, watching the sycamore leaves flickering in the summer breeze outside. But I would never be the same. It was the moment I seemingly grew up. The knowledge of my new grown-up self was bewildering to my little four- or five- or six-year-old mind. *How could I be grown when I was so little?* But the pain and the fear and the shame of what happened to me was so enormous that I *had* to be grown to carry it.

At the very same time, I felt stuck—fully grown and forever stuck. Stunted. To compensate, I shoved the hurting and broken little girl who lived inside me waaaaaay into the dark attic corners of my mind, and I tried to ignore her. I attempted to shame her away. I cursed at her. And I yelled at her. I told her she was ugly and fat and stupid and weak. I told her if anyone knew the truth, they would probably just leave, and she would be alone. Abandoned. Forgotten. To keep her quiet there in the corner, I told her she was worthless. And I tried to help her earn people's love through accomplishments. Because . . . *maybe if we were somehow good enough?* But it never worked. "Goodness" never made the hurting little girl disappear.

Shame never could make me well.

No matter what I did, that small girl was always there, crouched in the corner. She peered out at me from the shadows from time to time with desperate eyes, pleading, *Is it okay now? Are we okay? Did I do all right? Am I lovable?* She simply wanted my love.

It took me nearly forty years. But I am learning, now, to love her.

Focus on Healing

Of course, we would always like to know why—*Why did this happen?* But really, there is no why. It just . . . did. We hope to make our hurt disappear, but hurt can't disintegrate into thin air. It's simply there. We want to run and hide, but the pain finds us. We try to shame it away by binging or raging or hiding or sleeping. We attempt to cover it up with drugs or alcohol or meaningless sloppy sex or even a loud, boisterous personality and black-gauge earrings and scads of colorful tattoos. We eat or restrict. We exercise or work or strive or achieve. We acquire a lengthy list of bright and shiny accomplishments and fancy titles like "Dr. Albertson" in a seemingly perfect life, desperately hoping to be loved. But then when we inevitably fail, we chastise ourselves mercilessly. We might even dig into our arms until they bleed mostly because we just want to feel . . . something. And if we could peel back all the layers to the core of what's hiding inside, we would discover the hurt again. Seemingly fresh and new.

We've been taught by the world that people who are hurt or poor or fat or lost or incarcerated must lack self-control. We don't want to be one of *those* people. So, instead we let our nasty inner critic hold our hurting insides hostage and attempt to manhandle our unruly parts and our ugly pasts into behaving. We try to control all our hurt and pain and trauma with ongoing and relentless shame.

Then to add insult to our own self-injury, sometimes the "wellness" industry chimes in and sells us something to "help."

Countless new programs or diets or exercise regimens or supplements or self-help books promise to boost our willpower and instill self-discipline, often with even more shame: *No pain, no gain. Failure is NOT an option. Success is a decision. Now, get out there and kick some ass! Feel great! You really can crush all your goals!*

Such self-inflicted, shame-*based* "*health*" behaviors may include

- Damaging language or internal verbal abuse
- Self-exclusion from pleasurable activities like eating or relaxing
- Dietary restriction of entire food groups (remember "no carbs" is disordered eating)
- Empty promises or threats for "misbehavior"
- Embarrassment and self-humiliation
- Constant comparison to others
- Intimidation and harsh self-criticism
- Even self-harm

Unfortunately, the harder we try to rid ourselves of hurtful memories, bad thoughts, or negative emotions using shame, the stronger they become. Our bodies and souls simply do not respond positively to shame. Instead, shame-based behaviors may push us into maladaptive coping strategies like alcohol or drugs, an increased likelihood of depression or anxiety, poor job performance, broken relationships, people-pleasing tendencies, increased aggression, disordered eating, rage, violence, cutting and self-harm, and even a tendency toward suicidal thinking.

Trauma *changes* us. That's true. But we can't ignore it any longer. Our pain and trauma need attention more than anything else, and instead of attempting to control our hurt with shame, there is something much more productive we can do.

207

What we (and the hurting inner children within us) need instead of shame is compassion. We need deep understanding. And love. Without love, the cycle of trauma simply passes on in one form or another from human to human to human. Love is the path toward breaking the cycle of trauma toward resiliency and fierce, true healing—the ongoing healing we will navigate for a lifetime. We *need* this healing. So, what do we do?

Steps toward love-based healing

1. **Acknowledge where harm or injury has occurred.** Be brave. Look honestly at your past and take a vulnerable inventory. Tell the truth about where wrongdoings have occurred and about your feelings in response. Telling the truth has a way of dispersing things, of blowing the white fluff away from the stem so you can watch it dance in the breeze. You will likely process past harm best if you can work closely with a therapist specifically trained to treat trauma.

2. **Respond to your emotions with self-compassion and empathy.** Dr. Hillary McBride suggests responding to yourself with words of kindness like "of course." *Of course* you are struggling. *Of course* you have pain and shame centered around that particular event. It was hurtful and scary, so *of course* you will need time and help in order to heal. It is normal and okay that you feel this way. *Of course* you do![2]

3. **Be patient.** Foster a sense of open-minded curiosity about your body, your feelings and emotions, your interests and talents, your relationships, your growth, and your future possibilities. Understand that healing through trauma takes time—forever, even—and let yourself be proud of your progress toward breaking unhealthy cycles.

4. **Seek secure and loving relationships with deep, meaningful connections.** Learn to be close with others so you can

move into compassionate relationship with yourself. It doesn't take many; just a few or even one safe, loving relationship can remind you that you are not alone and you are worthy of love and care. We'll talk more about the team God sends to help us along the way in chapter 15.

5. **Restore trust and safety with your Self by responding with encouragement, warmth, and support.** Accounting for what happened in your life and who and why you are the way you are, where you've been hurt, how you've succeeded or failed in your attempts at healing, plus all the ways you are prioritizing your own health and care and safety moving forward demonstrates your incredible *resilience*. This actionable work is the path toward becoming a whole and healthy individual you can trust—the making of your true and trustworthy Self.

When I met Krystal, I was a PRN provider. And though I never treated her again as a patient, it was the beginning of real, honest, and secure treatment for her with a psychiatrist and a therapist and additional medications for support. I still think of her often. I pray for her often. And I honor the small hurting child within her by encouraging the small hurting child within myself to grow. To pursue change and love and healing. To choose resilience. Every day I practice reaching *beyond the pain* of trauma toward a life filled with fierce self-compassion. A life of tender mercy and hope and resiliency. A life with the stunning, God-given capacity to endure. A true and beautiful life filled to the brim with love.

Trauma changes us, it's true. But *love* is how we heal.

14

SEASONS OF HEALING

How to Live in Your Season

Recently, a dear friend called to tell me the devastating news that her grown daughter is an addict and she's struggling. My friend knew, of course. But the extent to which her daughter has been struggling only recently came to light because she lost both a job and a boyfriend of several years within the same week due to her drug abuse. Now the fallout looms large.

Her daughter tried cutting back. She tried therapy off and on. She tried medication for depression. But nothing seems to help. My friend is desperate to talk her daughter into going to a more intensive inpatient drug rehab facility, but nothing works. Her daughter won't listen.

This very dear friend called me because she knows my husband was in and out of rehab years ago, and now he's been in recovery for over fifteen years. She called me because she knows I am basically incapable of small talk and will gladly take the deep dive into all the devastating parts of life right along beside her. She called me because she knew I wouldn't offer any advice and would simply respond with something like, "Ugh. I'm sorry. Life can be so hard. I love you." She called me because for just a little while she was hoping to feel less alone.

I tried very hard to listen.

Of course, a tiny part of me wanted to suggest she go to Al-anon and get a sponsor and work the twelve steps. I also considered ordering a few books from the "approved Al-anon literature" list to send to her, maybe a daily devotional or the Big Book. And I very much wanted to suggest daily self-care. But somehow, miraculously, I bit my tongue and managed to keep my advice to myself as I said, "Ugh. I'm sorry. Life can be so hard. I love you."

Apparently, my friend's daughter is one of those high-functioning addicts, meaning she manages to hold a job (or at the very least, a job here or there) and pays off most of her bills and carries on like a mostly normal and functioning member of society. Except then she occasionally drinks herself into oblivion and regularly takes prescription painkillers that she buys illegally off the internet so that her mind is only ever semi-present in the current moment and mostly floating in a cloud of narcotics. My friend is expectedly devastated.

Life really can be *so* hard.

What we want most for our children is simple, really. We hope they will have passion. We hope they will find a few fulfilling relationships and some purposeful work. We hope that occasionally in the middle of life they will stumble upon a bit of everyday, ordinary joy. We want our children to *live*, and my friend's precious daughter is only half living.

Not long after I hung up the phone with my friend, I came upon an article about how "life can be good again" after something devastating happens. The writer of the article had a young child who suffered from an aggressive form of cancer, and the treatments and aftermath of that diagnosis sent the writer into a tailspin, knocking her completely off her feet for a while. She didn't think she'd ever be able to call life "good" again.

211

Then, miraculously, her child was healed. And apparently the writer of the article was changed for the better by the whole ordeal. She wrote this encouraging article to offer help and support for those who are struggling. She promised with her story that life can be good again after devastation. That life is *better* even because of our terrible pain.

I thought hard about my friend from our old neighborhood and her half-living daughter.

Then I thought about all the people whose children *don't* get better from their aggressive forms of cancer. The people who lose their precious, beloved children. The people who suffer through unbearable losses and unthinkable traumas in life—all manner of abuse, loss of loved ones, infidelity, deep betrayal, messy divorces, childhood hurts and resulting complex post-traumatic stress, chronic illnesses, life-threatening diseases, or even . . . watching your daughter be sucked into the depths of addiction unable to surface from its clutches. The people who will not, in fact, be *better* because of their terrible pain.

I texted my friend with the alcohol- and drug-addicted daughter a link to the article along with an eye-rolling emoji. She sent a laughing face in reply and texted back, *Why do people write crap like this?* It truly made me LOL.

Can life ever truly be *good* again? I'm not sure. But I do know life happens in seasons. It says so right there in Ecclesiastes, right?

> There is a time for everything,
>   and a season for every activity under the heavens:
> a time to be born and a time to die,
> a time to plant and a time to uproot,
> a time to kill and a time to heal,
> a time to tear down and a time to build,
> a time to weep and a time to laugh,
> a time to mourn and a time to dance,
> a time to scatter stones and a time to gather them,
> a time to embrace and a time to refrain from embracing,

> a time to search and a time to give up,
> a time to keep and a time to throw away,
> a time to tear and a time to mend,
> a time to be silent and a time to speak,
> a time to love and a time to hate,
> a time for war and a time for peace.
>
> —Ecclesiastes 3:1–8

God truly can make everything beautiful *in its time*, but we simply can't do our lives all at once. There is a time for all of it because life happens in seasons.

Maybe you're personally in a season of thriving. And every day you're getting your kids up and off to school then jumping into your size-four pants and grabbing a fruit smoothie with a scoop of protein before heading off to work, where you recently celebrated a promotion because there, too, you're absolutely nailing it. Maybe you are, in fact, in a season of kicking ass and crushing goals. Please know, I'm happy for you. I am. I'm over here cheering!

Or maybe, like me, you're in a season of healing. And every day you're waking up with deep theological questions pelting your mind and you're digging into all the reasons why you are the way you are and where you've been hurt and what you need—like rest and deep connection and exercise (with weight training as well as flexibility and balance training) and psychotherapy and a new set of clothes that you feel good in because they actually fit rather than the old sizes you've been squeezing yourself into—hoping to become a truer and more beautiful version of you. Maybe you are in a season of searching for mercy and meaning and grace in this one precious, beautiful life.

Or maybe right now you're in a season of surviving terrible pain. And every day you're rolling over trying not to scream into your pillow because the sun has risen again, and you must face another horrible, gut-wrenching day. Perhaps the pain you're feeling right now feels completely unsurvivable. And the idea of "flexibility and balance training" and "rest or deep connection" makes you want to tear out your hair and rip off your clothes and run into the middle of the street because *what the hell??? Why does it matter??? And why in God's name does this wretched life have to hurt SO MUCH???* But then mostly because of guilt and what our culture tells you about self-care, you make a fruit smoothie and drag yourself off to your job (which you despise) instead. Please believe me when I say, I'm sorry. Life can be so hard. And I love you.

A few years ago, I took care of a patient who was emerging from a season of life just like that—a season of deep and terrible pain that she barely survived.

Like clockwork, Elaine came to see me for a check-up every six months. I knew her as a woman in her late forties with elevated blood pressure, borderline-controlled type 2 diabetes, moderate depression, and obesity managed on a few daily medications who came for regular maintenance appointments and blood work. I also knew her to be kind and bright, quiet and sarcastic, incredibly beautiful, and often, wickedly funny. In our visits over those few years, Elaine shared bits and pieces of her story with me, and it was clear that she hadn't had a wonderful life. In fact, her life was often atrocious.

She grew up in an abusive home with a father who drank too much in the evenings after his construction work and often treated her mother terribly. He wasn't physically abusive to the children, but they all lived in fear of his emotional abuse and violent nature toward their mother.

Elaine's childhood pain and abuse brought more pain and more abuse when she eventually married an equally heinous man. He was even more angry and violent and abusive than her father had been, especially when he spent the evening drinking alcohol. And for over a decade, Elaine had attempted to free both herself and her daughter from their abusive home.

Life was *hard*, but Elaine was strong. She was an amazing mother. She was incredibly resourceful and intelligent, and through it all, she never lost hope. Though she wasn't sure she could financially afford to be a single mother on the meager salary she earned as a receptionist at a flooring store, eventually Elaine fled with her daughter. They left the abuse and the drinking and the violence and the pain, and they began the lifelong journey of restoration and repair.

Now Elaine tells the story of her childhood and married past with a mixture of deep sadness and courageous pride. None of it was what she wanted for her life or for her one beautiful daughter's childhood, and yet she is here. She did the best she could do with the tools available to her at the time, and she is still standing. Elaine is continuing to heal.

During every visit I had with Elaine, I reviewed her blood pressure and listened to her heart and lungs. I examined her legs for edema and asked about side effects from her medications. I refilled her prescriptions and ordered blood work to make sure her diabetes was under adequate control and her kidneys were functioning well and her cholesterol was at goal. I encouraged yearly maintenance exams and all the necessary preventative care.

We talked about coping skills and her mood and anxiety levels as well as any other long-term effects. We discussed how the daily medication she took for depressive symptoms seemed to be helping. I applauded her continued efforts to pursue counseling as a tool on her path to healing. And though I encouraged healthy lifestyle changes—limiting processed foods, eating plenty of vegetables, proteins, and whole grains, moving her body daily to relieve stress—I never did give her a lecture on the importance of weight loss and treating her medical problems by focusing on her obesity. I could not bear to give her a list of ways she could do better. I would not foist upon her that endless striving to be *better*, somehow, so she could "kick ass" or "crush goals" or be more admired by the world as a pinnacle of health and wellness.

Elaine was living in a season of safety and security and precarious courage and beauty, which meant she was healing in her own

215

way. On her own time. Elaine was simply . . . amazing. And one afternoon when I opened the exam-room door, I was confronted with Elaine's sparkling eyes.

"Dr. Albertson, I gotta tell you what we did!"

Perching on my little round doctor's stool, I leaned toward her. I could barely wait. "What? What did you do?"

"Well, me and Melissa, we've been saving for years, now. Plus, you know, Melissa *loves* to fish. She'd fish every weekend if she could!"

Then she paused for dramatic effect, eyes still sparkling.

"Well . . . we bought a camper!" she cried, erupting into laughter. "Can you believe it? We didn't even know if the old thing could run!"

Delighted, she told me all about their old, broken-down camper and every summer weekend they spent camping together at various campgrounds. Meeting people and fishing and eating hot dogs and s'mores.

"Yeah, it's great. We just pack up a bunch of food in a cooler, and I sit in my lawn chair in the sun and watch her fish. She loves it!"

Elaine's eyes danced. It was clear she loved this time with her little healing family.

And I very much loved seeing her face filled with the pride of really living a life on her own terms. Elaine was more than surviving. With elevated blood pressure, type 2 diabetes, depression, obesity, a dreadful past, and the sheer delight of an old, broken-down camper beside the daughter she loves, Elaine was *thriving*. In a million small ways day after day, she is a little bit happy and a little bit sad and extremely proud of her one precious, beautiful life *exactly as it is*. And really, what could be *better* than that?

Digging Deeper into Seasons

Our brains are designed to keep us safe. As we discussed in chapter 3, we are *wired* for safety, and any danger or threats to our well-being will kick our brains into survival mode, triggering the stress response toward fight, flight, or freeze. We also already discussed that chronic stress affects the body, especially the capital-T trauma type of stress we may carry due to childhood adversity or deep losses in adulthood. The hurts we experience throughout life can begin to rewire our biological systems, and we may come to feel as if there are constant threats to our basic needs, resources, and sense of safety.

As a result, our overactive stress response may have a very low threshold for triggering the physiological cascade of hormones from the sympathetic nervous system, and our brains might consistently jump to conclusions about current potentially dangerous situations based on our conditioning from the past. Even simple healthy steps like changing our diet or getting into a regular exercise program or connecting with a friend in vulnerable ways or visiting the doctor for an annual exam can overwhelm our nervous systems, setting off the stress cascade like a major attack on our safety.

This is why sometimes, for example, though I truly believe quitting smoking is imperative for health and longevity since it is a risk factor for almost every chronic illness, I *don't* encourage smoking cessation for every patient. Instead, we decide together whether quitting right now is the right time. If there's too much else going on—a divorce, grief from a recent death, some other huge life stressor—we wait and circle back when perhaps things quiet down so that smoking cessation has the most chance of success. Yes, I want everyone to quit smoking. But sometimes we simply need to find the right time and season.

Our bodies have only so much bandwidth, only so much energy and mental capacity to deal with whatever the day throws our way. And sometimes it is okay to admit that *safety* is top priority today rather than achieving some prescribed level of "ideal" health, even in the face of chronic illness like elevated blood pressure, borderline-controlled type 2 diabetes, depression, or the complicating factor of obesity, as it was for Elaine.

Sometimes gentleness is the best healing practice for today.

Focus on Healing

So, what do we do? How do we know? Is there any way to evaluate our readiness for change?[1] How can we live *fully* in our current season? And how do we adjust our expectations and priorities to match our capacity for change in our current season of healing?

Here are a few questions to ask yourself about change in your current season

1. What is the motivation behind your desire to change? Are *you* the driver? Or is your desire to change related to the expectations of the larger cultural ideal?

2. Considering your current life situation and general day-to-day capacity, how much bandwidth do you have to allocate toward change?

3. What is the need behind this change—is this particular change important to your health? Or safety? Will it make a difference in your comfort? Or healing? Or long-term health?

4. Can this change be maintained over time? Or will you be riding the yo-yo, ending up worse than where you started?

5. How can you begin now to create an actionable plan with the least possibility for setbacks or relapse and the greatest chance for long-term commitment?

Britt Frank is a licensed psychotherapist, trauma specialist, and the author of *The Science of Stuck* who introduced the concept of "micro-yesses" to help reassure a jumpy nervous system (which has been conditioned to overreact because of previous traumas) that you will keep your word to YOU. Micro-yesses are a way to reassure yourself that *you* have *your* best interest and continued safety at heart. And micro-yesses allow us to match our capacity for change with our current season of healing. A micro-yes is smaller than a small step. It's smaller than a baby step. A micro-yes is the smallest possible thing you can do without your nervous system going into fight/flight/freeze.[2]

We can give micro-yesses by noticing what we need, then taking steps toward meeting that need:

- We give micro-yesses by waking up every morning around the same time, eating breakfast, getting dressed, brushing our teeth, greeting the day with love, and heading out the door toward whatever we're trying to accomplish that day.
- We give micro-yesses by acknowledging our immediate needs like stopping for the restroom when we feel the urge or noticing our small bodily cues of hunger, loneliness, warmth or chilliness, boredom, or tiredness, then taking the next small step toward alleviating that discomfort.
- We give micro-yesses when we buy a pack of orange gum from the store or wrap ourselves in a blanket straight from the dryer, simply because it tastes good or feels warm and makes us remember we are deeply and fully loved by our Creator.

With tiny, incremental steps we cross what may be a rickety bridge toward healing by continuing to show up for ourselves in thousands of small ways day after day after day, instilling a deep sense of safety, love, and trust. *In ourselves.*

We can start incorporating micro-yesses with one or two very small, easily available choices *right now* that will move us forward toward better health and healing. Meaning, instead of committing yourself to drinking sixty-four ounces of water every day because drinking water is good for you and you definitely drink too much soda, you can simply decide to have *one glass of water right now.* Or instead of signing up for a half-marathon and writing out a lengthy exercise schedule that has you waking up at 5:00 a.m. six days a week and adding at least a mile or two to each week's running routine, you can choose to head out for *a ten-minute walk right now*. If it's your smoking habit you want to change, maybe you can start by cutting down on smoking or find a friend to quit with or take up walking as a substitute during your smoke breaks at work.

Understanding your current season and your current bandwidth and capacity for health and healing, then practicing teeny tiny micro-yesses multiple times throughout the day can bring a feeling of safety and security and trust within yourself to move you toward true inner healing. In the middle of life's difficulties and pain, we simply take one tiny micro-yes toward love at a time.

※ ※ ※ ※

My friend with the drug- and alcohol-addicted daughter called the other day to report that little has changed. Her daughter continues to choose not to go to rehab and, instead, suffers along day after day smacked out of her mind on prescription painkillers she orders illegally off the internet, only half-living the fleeting moments of her one precious, beautiful life. My friend told me how deeply it hurts to watch her daughter suffer. How painful it is for her momma heart. How desperately she wants to help. And how unbearable it feels to detach from her daughter's decisions and half-living lifestyle, and simply love her daughter anyway.

I listened.

I said, "Ugh. I'm sorry. Life can be so hard. I love you." Then I added, "You know, you're doing *so* beautifully under some very terrible circumstances. It isn't fair. And I'm proud of you."

There was a silence on the other end of the line, then she sniffed a little and told me something new.

She told me her daughter came for dinner on Sunday, and she seemed clear-headed for the first time in a long time. My friend told me how the two chatted and recalled a few precious memories and laughed. And how they played a few rounds of cards together as a family before her daughter went back to her apartment for the night (possibly to get smacked out of her mind). My friend told me it was a beautiful evening. And though she may never get what she wants—a beautiful life for her one beautiful daughter that is free from mind-altering substances and filled with passion and connection and purpose and even a bit of everyday, ordinary joy—she realized that beauty can occasionally pierce through the hard. And life can sometimes feel semi-okay again.

I thought about Elaine and her daughter going fishing with their camper. I thought about Maureen and her son playing Scrabble at the hospital together. I thought about Krystal and her patients in the evening care respite program. I thought about how for some of us it is entirely possible that life may never be "good" again. Not really. But it *can* be semi-okay.

And perhaps knowing this, bits of passion or connection, small fragments of purpose, and even tiny moments of joy will push their way through the cracks that have formed in our hearts in response to life's pain and devastation. Perhaps with small steps and micro-yesses, we might discover beauty and healing in a season of life that is mostly (or at least sometimes) semi-okay.

Semi-okay can be a miracle.

15

BUILDING A TEAM

One of my children once wrote something very sad in his school journal. It was the kind of devastating admission the principal calls home about. The kind of thing you begin making frantic calls to set up therapy appointments about; the kind that leaves you gripping your chest, heaving great wheezing breaths, replaying all the millions of ways you've dropped the ball as a mother and failed your beloved child.

At the end of that year after lots of discussions and therapy, his teacher—the sort of amazing teacher who brings a loving presence to the classroom and truly understands and cares about children (especially during the unfortunate years of early adolescence)—wrote a note in the back of my child's yearbook:

> *You are a born leader; however, that doesn't mean you need to carry all the heavy stuff by yourself. Don't forget to use your team. They are there to help you.*
>
> *From, Your Teammate*

I wish I had known this information in elementary school. I wish I had learned it by the time I entered college or medical school or during early motherhood or on those desperately lonely days when my husband was on drugs and in and out of rehab. Frankly, I wish I could always remember it now. I worry that so many of us are dying of loneliness.

When we moved to our first little house on Poppleton Street near the hospital where I completed my medical training, my husband was desperately hooked on drugs. He was *always* either high on drugs, sleeping off his last high, or waiting impatiently to get high again. He simply couldn't bear to be sober in his own life. And for the longest time I fumbled along helplessly beside him.

The Poppleton House, as we now call it, was our first home. It was a postage-stamp-sized house with crisp white paint, black shutters, and a bright red front door. For weeks before we moved into that little house, I'd do a drive-by viewing before heading to the hospital for a seemingly endless call shift. I'd roll down my window in the morning darkness and poke my nose outside to smell the fresh, wet dirt bursting to life in spring and stare, letting my mind wander. I could barely wait to start our family there. I could barely wait to start a whole new life there. I could barely wait for my real life to begin. And it seemed this little house had been waiting for me, too. Our first baby, Isaiah, was born *exactly* thirty-nine weeks and four days after our move-in day (which seems meaningful if you know he came three days early and you stop to do the math).

I cried a lot in that house. And we fought a lot. I watched my husband stumble through his life, hands shaking. I watched him sink further away from me into the pit of addiction. There was angry shouting and silent desperation and terrible, debilitating sadness. But still, I planted morning glories out back along the fence, where every morning those purple blossoms opened wide and stretched toward the sun in the same way we turn our faces toward the light and stretch toward grace.

I became a mother in that home. I changed tiny diapers and learned to breastfeed and rocked our new baby quietly in my green chair. And I distinctly remember the day I switched from holding a small, swaddled baby tenderly in my arms to settling his chubby diapered bottom solidly on my hip and thinking, *Oh my God, I have waited my whole life for this.* I didn't yet know that I would have a baby or toddler fixed delightfully to that hip for the next fifteen years. It was the saddest time I can remember. Yet it was the happiest I had ever been. In that little house on Poppleton Street I learned the two—pain and joy—can coexist. One feeling made that much stronger because of the other. Pain and joy. Joy and pain.

I loved the squeaks and groans of those original hardwood floors, the wide sweeping arches separating the small rooms, the dainty glass doorknobs, and that wide brick fireplace with the long white mantle. I loved the collective *history* I felt in that space. And I spent hours perched on the cracked cement steps of our front porch, where towering cottonwood trees arched overhead, lining the street. From there, I watched my life change as I observed my children play and grow.

When Isaiah was a baby, I often spread a blanket on the tiny stretch of lawn beneath the sweeping branches of those trees so the two of us could lie together watching the limbs dance, sunlight dappling through the leaves. Two years later when his little brother, Eli, joined the mix, I suddenly had two little boys running barefoot on the lawn, laughing and chasing, their pudgy feet slapping against the cement of the sidewalk. The late-afternoon summer sun pierced through those cottonwood branches overhead, illuminating fluffs of white cotton that floated gently on the breeze and landed on my boys' fuzzy blond heads. I watched it all from the crumbling steps of our porch.

My life had been reduced to rubble by my husband's worsening addiction and our failing marriage, by the realities of early motherhood with two little boys beside a demanding job at the hospital that leeched away any remainder of my energy and time. Yet somehow, those towering cottonwoods above reassured me that ninety years prior another family had lived in this very same place. That another woman had planted those giant cottonwood trees *just* for my children to pad beneath on bare feet. The knowledge

224

of her made me feel less afraid and alone. Pain and joy. Joy and pain. This is how we live, but we don't have to do it alone.

God builds us a team.

Our teammates help us understand who we are and fill our deepest needs: to be seen, to be heard, to find meaning in our lives, to wake up and grow and belong to those who love and care for us. They show us what community and friendship feel like. And they are just a teeny part of this treacherous life that can begin to fill the God-sized hole in our hearts because they are gifts sent directly *from* God. They teach us what it means to be fully loved, in Him.

It was during that sad and joy-filled time in my life that I met Anne—a beacon of light and hope in a world marked by pain and loss and grief and bittersweet sadness, a world I couldn't possibly control no matter how many times I tried.

The blunt bob cut of Anne's silver hair grazed the shoulders of her scrub top, which she always paired with soft, worn cardigans and running shoes (comfortable footwear was a must for Anne). Her eyes were hazel-blue and kind; they dazzled with kindness. I think that's what I liked about her most—the way her eyes and her crow's feet and her smile and her smart, gray bob cut and the tone of her voice and her dry humor and her whole aura just *exuded* kindness.

Anne had a face of love.

I worked with Anne, a part-time nurse practitioner, at our downtown sexually transmitted disease (STD) clinic on Monday, Wednesday, and Friday evenings during residency. She managed the clinic after her day job, working three weeks on followed by one week off. And sometimes during "off" weeks when her two high-school-aged children were with their dad, Anne went to stay with a friend in California, where she also volunteered at a foot clinic adjacent to a homeless shelter.

Anne shared that most afternoons in California, she walked the beach and let the surf spill up over her toes in the sand. Her eyes twinkled with excitement as she described it. Then she explained that in her downtime, she worked in the nearby homeless shelter washing people's feet. She used soap and warm water in a basin to remove dirt or blood or dry skin. Then she applied foot cream or triple-antibiotic ointment, bandaged up cuts, trimmed and filed toenails, and neatly dressed the worn, cracked feet of people experiencing homelessness with fresh pairs of soft, white socks.

I admired the way Anne spoke honestly about life, about *all* of it—about her divorce, her wandering college-aged children, the homeless shelter where she volunteered, her messy patients with their ailments and their profane language and their stories about drug use or prostitution plus their children and families and their current struggles. She didn't condone and she didn't condemn; she only treated and helped. She simply loved and served.

During those evening STD clinics, side by side, Anne and I took histories and collected swabs or urine specimens, then we handed out antibiotic pills or powder to mix into miniature white Dixie cups of water for patients to swallow down on the spot. We were incredibly efficient, and during each four-hour clinic, up to twenty or thirty, even forty patients shuffled through. And this nurse practitioner oversaw it all—gruff men with colorful language, women with pudgy babies perched on their hips or toddlers grabbing at their knees, teenagers waving long, wildly painted fake fingernails and sporting terrible cases of Chlamydia. Anne smiled and laughed, asked them questions, pinched their babies' thighs, and doled out rounds of antibiotics along with plenty of hugs.

One Wednesday evening before Thanksgiving, I caught a few lines of Anne's one-sided phone conversation with her youngest daughter. She'd been excited throughout clinic over her college-aged kids returning home for the long weekend. Now her voice was joyful as she hooked the phone under one ear while piling completed charts neatly on the corner of her desk.

"I don't know what I'm making. Just pull some hamburger out of the freezer and get it started, okay? We'll figure it out when I get home."

She paused. "What? Oh my, he said *that*?" Then she laughed. "What a jackass! That sucks, sweetheart. You must've had a rough day. Let's talk more about it tonight."

Another pause. Then a tiny squeal. "Yes! They're on their way! Nine o'clock. I can't wait either. Love you, hon. See you in a bit."

I stared. I was simply mesmerized by this woman's way with people—with her own children and *all* of God's children. There was something different about her, something about the kindness in her eyes. She wasn't afraid of anyone's lives or their stories. She simply walked along beside whoever crossed her path, helping where she could. I learned so much from the evenings I spent working side by side in the clinic with Anne.

Months later at my regular Sunday morning Al-Anon group, shortly after my husband completed his stay in the three-quarter-way house, a new face appeared behind the podium claiming a turn to speak. I hadn't seen her since I'd fulfilled the graduation requirement for shifts in the STD clinic. And I almost didn't recognize Anne without those navy scrubs. But she'd thrown the same tattered cardigan over a T-shirt with jeans, and her kind, hazel-blue eyes were unchanged.

"This isn't my normal group," she began. "But I have a plane to catch to California later this afternoon, and I wanted to join a quick meeting before I left. I've been in Al-Anon rooms a *very* long time. And I have a long and awful story to tell—an ex-husband with a terrible drinking problem, a very messy divorce. Plus, now my children are growing and leaving home. And many days I have no idea what I'm doing as a mother, let alone how I'll pay for any of it. But that's not what I want to share today."

I sucked in my breath, still not quite sure it was her. Not quite sure I was allowed to hear the intimate details of this woman's life when what I knew to this point was her professional life as a nurse practitioner treating patients. But she caught my eye and winked.

"I've been taking these trips to California off and on this year to see my friend who is dying from cancer. And in my downtime, I volunteer at a foot clinic in a shelter for people experiencing home-lessness. I wash people's feet." She smiled, and her eyes glanced out the leaded-glass window to the bare trees outside before she continued.

"During my last visit, this man I've treated before showed up, say-ing he wished he could repay me . . ." Her voice trailed away as she puffed out a slow breath through pursed lips and wiped away tears.

"He asked if we could switch seats . . . and he . . . he proceeded to wash my feet." She stopped, then, and looked down at her hands, mouth quivering. "He washed *my* feet."

"I guess what I'm saying is, I was so lonely for so long. Every-thing felt terrible and broken. I was so lost. I didn't know if life would ever get better. If I would ever find healing, you know? And I just . . . I don't know. I started showing up for life. Like *really* living. And then this man—you should've seen the condition of his hands." She hesitated. "He washed *my* feet."

Then she stopped. Her eyes scanned the room before her gaze settled on my face, and she smiled wide. "I just felt like that's the story I wanted to share today. Thank you."

The people I admire most are those who've walked through the pit, who've trudged their way through the muck and mire and somehow clawed their way through to the other side. Changed. The people who have earned every bit of their healing and come out the other side with a whole new understanding of life and people and love—a little healthier, a little more tender, a little more wholehearted, a little more . . . whole. The people who turn and stretch out a hand from the other side, hoping to steady you as you claw your way through your own pit. People like Anne who, unbeknownst to her, became the leader of my team.

❋ ❋ ❋ ❋

All my life God has been building me a team.

I had a handful of brilliant teachers growing up. People who changed me with just one small through-line of support. Ms.

Richey in fourth grade taught me that loving books the way we both did was extremely important. Mr. Hammond, my high school English teacher, scrawled with tiny red letters on my essays: *You are a beautiful and talented writer, Mikala.* And Mr. Oltmans gave me the only B I had ever received (in AP Calculus), perhaps the best lesson I learned in high school.

I can still hear my high school Spanish teacher, Mrs. Alberry, clapping and clicking her heels as she danced down the aisles of the classroom in a swishy skirt, "Tengo una cita con Anita a las oche de la noche!" Years later and well into her eighties, Mrs. Alberry began following my blog and commenting on every piece. We messaged each other back and forth, and one day she promised to send a copy of the book she'd written about her own life. But then she died. I cried, of course, but I was grateful we'd reconnected in those years before. A week later I discovered a big white envelope in my mailbox with Mrs. Alberry's name and address printed on the front. Hands shaking, I ripped open the envelope and her book landed in my lap. I turned to the inner flap to find a note scrawled in my beloved teacher's beautiful handwriting. She sent me a letter sent straight from heaven:

> *Never in my dreams did I see a student who endured a class of mine become so famous and outstanding in so many ways! Gracias for inspiring and remembering me!*
>
> *Love,*
> *Reina Maria*

In college, Dr. Kelter drew a gigantic smiley face in the 100% on my chemistry test (after the 54% on the previous test that I was sure meant I would fail out). And Dr. Hill saw me through the sadness behind the scenes of my medical school and residency years.

They were my teammates.

And now today, I have my kind and sober husband. My sister. My family. I have Jenny, who fields my phone calls nearly every single morning. I have Amy from my old neighborhood and Diana who lives twenty minutes away. I have the woman who smiles warmly at the store each time she beeps my groceries across the scanner. And the woman I wave to regularly when we cross paths on the walking trail. I have the kind doctor who prescribes my Lexapro. And my therapist. I have my neighbor Sharon. My aunts and cousins. And on top of *all* that, I have Emily and Amy and Mehr and Cassie and Angela, Jessica and Jenni and Angie and Michelle, Katie (a friend I picked up on an airplane), plus Amanda and Andrea and Rachel. And recently at a barbeque when someone asked—*Who is the friend you would call if you had to dispose of a body, no questions asked?*—the image of my friend Kari holding a shovel immediately came to mind. I have Kari, and I know she would simply start digging.

A Deeper Look at Healing through Connection

Studies show that social relationships are *crucial* to our long-term survival. Our connectedness to others has a powerful influence on our overall health and longevity, and a lack of social connection qualifies as a risk factor for premature mortality. Loneliness, in particular, is a leading predictor for all-cause mortality and contributes to cardiovascular disease, metabolic disorders, and mental illness.[1] Some evidence suggests that simply the *presence* of others—being close to other people and having regular human interaction—is just as essential as our deep, "quality" relationships, with potent effects on our health and well-being. In short, we simply need each other. So would you take a moment to consider your team?

Who instantly comes to mind?
Who haven't you considered a "team member" before?

Who changed you positively as a child?

Who were you impacted by that you never saw again?

Who do you still love dearly that you've had to let go of?

Who haven't you thought about for a while?

Who do you briefly pass every day with a wave and a smile?

Who has been there to support you through it all?

Who are the members of the team God designed specifically for YOU?

God sends people for our team to teach us how to know and love ourselves best as they hold us close, push us to grow, and lend us help along the way. And if we're very lucky, we find a select few who can tolerate our messes. These are the people who aren't afraid to turn their eyes *toward* our difficult emotions with kindness and compassion, listening quietly without offering solutions while our tender, broken hearts beat in their gentle hands. The people who allow us to be totally ourselves and share the most intimate parts of our lives. People we can trust. The ones who teach us how to love. These are the people who reach out a hand to steady us while we claw our way through the pit.

Here's a brief list of people you can consider for your team:

- Safe family members from both your nuclear and extended family units
- The influential teachers who taught you over the years
- Your trusted coworkers
- Your neighbors
- A pastor or priest and your friends from church
- Your healthcare providers—your doctor, nurses, your therapist, a dietician or personal trainer, your physical therapist
- Your friends (honestly, how would we *ever* survive without our friends?)

- Members of support groups or perhaps a recovery movement sponsor
- Your favorite writers, artists, and creatives
- This list is endless!!!

When life feels too hard, too much, or possibly unbearable, perhaps the only thing we can do is begin where we are. And I believe it's best if we stick together.

We need our teammates—even just a few—like we need air, water, food, and rest. Human connection is simply another form of nourishment, and without it, we will starve. Sometimes that connection means emotional support. Sometimes it's a meal delivered on a doorstep or a ride for one of our kids. Sometimes it's honest feedback or welcome accountability. Sometimes it's hard-to-hear truths. And sometimes it's a listening ear in the front seat of a friend's car in the Babies R Us parking lot while tears stream down your cheeks because your marriage is falling apart.

Of course, love and trust and friendship are nurtured best in relationships that are *reciprocal*, meaning the people on our team will give and receive in direct proportion to what we give and receive back. Not because our relationships are transactional, but because reciprocity makes us feel safe. *I feel safe when you share yourself and your stories, so now I can share myself and my stories with you.* Push and pull. Give and take. Back and forth. Yin and yang. In connected and healthy relationships, we simply take turns oscillating between the top and the bottom, the up and the down. And all the while, we walk along beside each other—holding hands, lending an ear, giving an encouraging smile, offering a pair of water wings to keep the other afloat.

Life is beautiful. Life is terrible. It's both. And sometimes our days can be so unbelievably hard we think we won't survive, but we don't have to do *any* of it alone because God builds us a team. Somehow, against all odds, we see each other through. We grab hands and claw our way up and out of the pit. And, as Ram Dass put it, we walk each other home.[2]

Don't forget to use your team. They are there to help you.

16

RE-MEMBERING YOUR *SELF*

I am sitting on the edge of a bed in the ICU at 5:00 a.m. My patient, Betty, has turned her pale face toward the hint of morning light tapping at the window, and I notice she looks calm. Peaceful. Serene. The fog of death she's been fighting against seems lifted for now (which I've come to understand is a sure sign the end is near), and her radiant eyes appear to be looking over the edge of something big, something new, something . . . grand. As if she is standing along the rim of the Grand Canyon for the very first time, taking in its wonder.

A beautiful woman by anyone's standards, Betty's particular beauty has nothing to do with her appearance (which, it turns out, is never a reliable or lasting marker for any of us). And until recently, she's been the pillar of health for an eighty-year-old. Feisty and active. A bit snarky and sweet. Whenever she visited me in clinic, she almost always wore sweatshirts with colorful, puff-painted scenes—autumn leaves blowing in the wind or snow falling onto a log cabin with smoke curling out of a little chimney—paired with elastic-waisted jeans and crisp white Ked sneakers. We spent half of each appointment talking about what she was growing in her garden or the lap blankets she stitched for the "old people" at the nursing home or whatever shenanigans my kids were up to or simply life in general (which meant my other patients were kept waiting, and I'd probably be working through lunch . . . again). But her sarcasm and wit were worth it.

Betty's only regular medical complaint was ongoing hip pain for which she eventually needed a hip replacement, and she passed her preoperative evaluation with flying colors. Her surgery went off without a hitch—there were no obvious complications—and the following day, the orthopedics team began making arrangements for discharge. Betty would go to a rehab facility for a week or so, then return home to her garden and her lap blankets and her life. That was the plan, until a day later when she was clinging to life in the ICU in florid congestive heart failure. I was devastated, wondering, *Where did I go wrong? Did I miss something? Did I screw up her IV fluids? Did I forget a medication or miss a dose? Did I overlook something important in her history? A lab value, maybe? How did I let this happen? And why in the world did I clear her for this elective surgery?* Betty had been perfectly healthy. Now . . . this.

I pored over her history, flipping with stubby-nailed fingers through the thin pages of her chart, reviewing the previous day's orders and meds and labs and vital signs, searching for any clue as to where I'd gone wrong. I was desperate for the answer. I simply could not accept the truth that pain and inexplicable sorrows await all of us. No. I wanted a solution. As the expert, I was supposed to diagnose the problem and fix it. *I am supposed to help make people's lives better and longer. I am supposed to offer the cure. After all, I spent a lot of money to go to school for a very long time.* But sometimes we can't help, not even a little bit. Sometimes we can't solve a life. Sometimes there is no cure. And sometimes sweet little eighty-year-old ladies suffer a silent heart attack during routine hip replacement surgery, and their fragile bodies simply can't recover.

Turns out, Jesus first introduced himself to me through other people. He'd been tapping me on the shoulder for years, inviting me to turn and follow Him, but mostly I ignored Him. I didn't intend to brush Him aside; I just wasn't listening. Too focused on my own plans for how my life should go. Too busy chasing the world and its promises for success and happiness and relevancy. Too busy hiding my faults and pain behind scholarships and awards and titles and what I imagined would create a beautiful life. I was simply too busy performing some cultural ideal to make much room for Jesus. It always felt like enough to imagine myself as His helper. I hoped to do something important with my life. Something necessary and possibly even noteworthy. *Because doesn't He need me, after all? To be His hands and feet?* And I'd done my best to help Betty until she fell ill.

In Al-Anon, I learned that H.O.P.E. is "hearing other people's experiences," and time and again, I've found this to be true. Al-Anon is where I learned to practice telling and receiving the Truth when all around my life was ripping at the seams. Then one day not long after that, I began working in the hospital, where I had the incredible privilege of witnessing the beauty of actually *being a human.* Of life. And death. Of stories and connection. Of failing bodies. And triumph. Of humanness. And the chance to stand so close to the ethereal.

What I've discovered over the years instead of any cure (and what I long to tell you now) is that right here in the middle, within the chaos of our broken bodies—in the disappointment and pain and shame and hormones and rage—*we are already living breathtakingly ordinary and meaningful lives.* Lives filled with beauty and empathy and humanity. Lives overflowing with hope. And love.

Ironically, I'm only now realizing that Jesus invites me to "help" much like I used to ask my toddlers if they wanted to "help" crack the eggs into the bowl when we mixed up a batch of chocolate chip cookies. I didn't really *need* their help, I just wanted to *be with them.* Jesus doesn't really *need* my help. But He loves me, and He simply wants to be with me. He asks all of us to serve the poor and the sick, the widowed and the orphaned, the imprisoned and the dying because that's where *He* is. He is there, so He asks us to be there. He just wants to be with us because He loves us. And His incredible, undeniable love is why I have written this book.

* * * *

Perhaps, desperate to find *the answer* to midlife, you picked up this book hoping I would give you a solution. I wonder if at this point in the story you'd like to raise your hand and ask, "But isn't there an easier way? Some essential oil I can use or an 'all natural' green powder I can add to my drink every morning to make me appear dewy and youthful? What about those new weight-loss drugs on the market? Should I take one? Do you recommend the 'mommy makeover surgery' and regular facial injections? Isn't there an app I can download on my phone with soft music or Catholic nuns chanting in Latin or something that will alleviate *all* my stress? I'm willing to pay."

Well, no.

I wish I had a secret formula I could let you in on. Some code word passed on to me from beautifully aging women who have managed to defy the typical aging process and remain stress-free and forever smooth and healthy and firm like Heidi Klum, who is obviously carrying a set of golden keys to unlock that magical door. But I don't. The process is pretty much the same for the rest of us. Every single woman I know—every woman I've cared for in clinic, my neighbors and aunts and relatives, my former classmates, my closest friends, the other mothers lining the soccer sidelines, every single one of us—is growing older. And along with these bodies that are now forty or fifty or sixty years old come quite a few bodily changes that are largely out of our control.

Plus, our bodies don't exist in a vacuum. *Life* happens, too.

Every over-forty woman alive is juggling the complexities of family care, career, relationships, and countless other responsibilities alongside the unattainable expectation that we can and should do it *all* while at the very same time our bodies are undergoing a revolution inside. It's a huge biological disruption that becomes so much more than simply hormonal changes because of the complex burden of *everything else* layered on top (like the threat of world war and a vet appointment for the dog at 9:00 a.m. and getting ten thousand steps and the school bake sale and an orthodontist appointment for the middle child at 3:00 p.m. and that earthquake in Turkey and back-to-back soccer practices this evening and our father's new cancer diagnosis and whether or not our dinner is sustainably sourced).

What we're feeling isn't exactly *normal*. It's a result of carrying the weight of the world. It's a bodily exhaustion deep in our bones caused by being worn down from life in a culture that is hostile to healthy living, both mentally and physically. What's demanded of middle-aged women is "beautiful" and "grateful" and "happy" and "firm." What's demanded is "youthful" and "thin" and "effortlessly sexy" and "joyful in motherhood," regardless of age or health or circumstances or *life*. And the pressure is lethal.

The problem that arises over and over again is that marketing promises us a solution to the unattainable picture of health and beauty we've been sold since childhood, so we tend to believe the picture exists. They tell us the answer is out there . . . somewhere. And we *want* help. We *want* the answers. We're so desperate for a quick fix that we turn to the "wellness" industry, where our pain points are exploited with promises of reprieve through some new product or "natural" supplement or miracle drug or extreme diet plan or sure-fire exercise routine. Hoping for a solution, we try them *all*:

- We starve our bodies of regular meals and entire food groups, attempting to work off any splurges to maintain a permanent calorie deficit, and we call it beauty or self-control or a "lifestyle."
- We deprive ourselves of healthy rest and much-needed sleep, and we call it grit.

- We push through long hours way past productivity with unfair treatment and unfair pay, and we call it partnership.
- We abandon hobbies and passions and friend relationships and personal interests, and we call it sacrifice.
- We chase the world's expectations and deplete ourselves for the benefit of *all* others—bending and stretching and breaking—being pulled in a thousand competing directions until we become completely dismembered, and we call it love.

I suppose now maybe you're saying, "Well, yes. That's probably true. I feel all of that. But is there any reason you haven't included a diet plan in this book to help me achieve my optimal weight during perimenopause?"

Sigh.

Yes, if you check appendix 5, you'll see I've referenced both the Dietary Approaches to Stop Hypertension (DASH) eating plan and the Mediterranean eating plan as two options for a well-balanced and heart-healthy diet you can follow. But I promise you'll never find what you're looking for that way.

What we *really* need is an undoing of the rules, of the stories we've been told, of the world's ridiculous expectations and the lies we've accumulated into overflowing garbage heaps in our minds. What we need is a re-membering of who we are and what we love and why we are here and what it really means to *live*. What we need in midlife is not another "life hack" for resilience or a diet for achieving our optimal weight, but a complete restructuring of our lives. We need a new and lasting definition for *beauty*, focusing on mental, spiritual, and physical health right here in the uniquely beautiful bodies we *actually* have.

My friend, this is your one precious, beautiful body. This is *you*. Your Self. Will you re-member her?

Maybe every morning when you shuffle into the bathroom to stare at your reflection in the mirror, you notice the lines framing your eyes. Yes, I know. I have them too. And yes, I suppose you could inject some of them away. But really, would you want to? Do you know how many laughs it took to create them? Think of the countless times you found delight in the endless gifts of this world and squinched up your eyes and laughed a great big belly laugh to leave all those lines behind. Day after day, month after month, year after year . . . laugh lines appearing like rings around the trunk of a tree. I bet if you count them, you have close to fifty.

And those sunspots on your cheeks? There are creams to lighten them. Sure. But those spots tell of hours playing in the sun as a child then years later pushing brand new babies in strollers on summer days or now cheering from your folding chair along the soccer sidelines or tending to the sea of flowers growing in your backyard. More evidence of moments spent turning your face toward the sun like morning glories planted along the fence.

Yes, your breasts may hang lower than they once did (and possibly a little unevenly like mine). But, really, would you trade a perkier pair for even one minute spent nursing your babies in the rocking chair or a single one of those milk-filled smiles?

Maybe your hips are wider now, too. Your hair growing streaks of gray. And maybe your over-forty tummy is softer and fuller than it once was, traced with silvery stretch marks from growth or scars from surgeries you've survived. These lines and marks and so-called imperfections are all just a reminder of a life well lived. A reminder of *years* of laughing and crying, of worry and sadness and struggle, of so very many grateful, happy smiles.

This beautiful, ordinary life you've been blessed with is evident right there on your body, etched in lines right there across your face. Perhaps instead of focusing on our physical flaws and imperfections and looking for solutions to hide them or take them away, we can simply notice the breathtaking beauty of everything we've overcome and all the *life* we carry in our looks.

I am so grateful for the opportunity to tell you about your body, about the lies of diet culture, about the hormonal changes of perimenopause, about mood disorders, about the marketing tricks of the "beauty and wellness" industry, about adult ADHD, about eating well(ish) and exercising for health and mobility rather than weight loss, about prioritizing sleep, about the gifts of connection with your team and the importance of practicing self-compassion and tenderness and mercy toward your fully human self. But what I long to tell you now is that there is just no *cure* for being human.

We *want* to be healed, of course. We want someone—a doctor or spouse or friend or new baby or boss handing out promotions or the latest marketing scheme or some all-natural healer—to come along with spackling compound and patch up the holes in our hearts before they wire our chests closed and stitch up the layers on top. But they can't. The stuff of the world cannot repair our hearts because our healing is an inside job. And anyway, as Leonard Cohen once told us, the cracks are how the light gets in.

Being human means we *will* experience pain and sadness and loss and change. We *will* feel lost and lonely and forgotten and alone. We *will* fail a thousand different times in a thousand different ways. And *all* of it will break our hearts. We are simply . . . human. And the pain of our humanness can hurt like hell, but it's necessary. It is the only way to crack our hearts open wide so we can begin to understand who we are, how to live and die, and why in the world we are here in the first place. The mess is simply proof that a *life* is being lived.

❋ ❋ ❋ ❋

In the ICU with Betty, the machines continue their faint whirring and beeping, and for a selfish moment as the early morning light streams in through the window, I wish she could tell me something important. I am tired of pretending. I am so weary. And I long to understand my life. My body. My purpose. I want to know if—right here at the end—she has finally figured out what it is all for. *What can she see there on the edge of eternity?* I am desperate for an answer. For meaning. For the . . . point. I want to shake her gently, *Betty, I don't understand my life. I'm not sure what I'm supposed to be doing here. And I have no idea how I'm supposed to fix any of it.*

But instead, I take her frail hand in mine and whisper, "Betty?"

She turns toward me, and her radiant eyes flicker with recognition, crinkling softly at the edges. The corners of her mouth curl into a faint smile, and the hospital bed becomes the whole world. I am surprised by the clarity of her face and the sturdiness of her presence, and I think, *Oh, hey Jesus. When did You get here?* I simply hadn't noticed Him before.

Then Betty pats my hand.

"Thank you for taking care of me, sweetheart," she says. "I love you."

And there it is. *Love.*

Love is the only thing we have left to offer in the face of life's inevitable pain and sadness and loss, and it's all we have when the rest of the world fades. What we have in the end is love, which means it's all we ever had in the first place. Not the stuff. Not the awards or accolades. Not the fancy house or perfect vacations. Not an arbitrary "goal weight" or a chiseled stomach. Not those perfect, matchy-matchy family photos plastered to the walls. Right here—amid the rubble—*we have love.*

When Betty died later that day, I waited in the hallway listening as her grown children held her hand and said their goodbyes.

"We're all here, Mom. All of us. We love you."

"It's okay. You were the *best* mom we could've asked for. We are so grateful. *So* grateful."

"It's okay to go. Dad is there waiting for you. We're okay, Mom. We'll be okay. Go to him."

"We love you!"

"We love you, Mom."

She held on for a few minutes more, then she simply . . . went. It took my breath away.

That's the thing about love. It makes us notice life's incredible beauty *right where it is*—in butterflies or ladybug larvae with those inside-out orange spots, in swirls of blue and purple clouds before a rain, in the smile of a friend's face across the table or a familiar voice on the other end of the line, in wildflowers of yellow and purple and orange along our favorite hiking path, in chubby baby legs with perfect pink toes, in cracked and work-worn hands, in the smell of cinnamon rising from the rolls in the oven, in the crow's feet framing our eyes after years of laughter and turning our faces toward the sun, in those very last beloved and heart-wrenching goodbyes.

Love is there. Waiting. Love is here. Now. Without any conditions or limits, love will never go away. It can *never* leave us. And somehow, some way . . . this eternal love takes the pressure off so that every morning we can wake up and look around at our Self and our imperfect body and this beautifully wretched life and decide it's not exactly what we had in mind, but it will do.

Yes, I *want* health and healing for you. I want you to live a long and meaningful life overflowing with passion and purpose. I want to help you find treatment options for your changing hormones and sleep issues or anxiety, for your disordered eating, your thyroid, or your focus. I care so much for your well-being. I truly want to help you be as healthy as possible for as long as humanly possible. And I want to offer you a path toward healing the one precious, beautiful body you *actually* have.

This book really is everything I wish I could tell you . . .

But if I had to choose—if I could tell you just one thing—it's that you are LOVED. *You are loved, loved, loved.* And love is the magical, ordinary revolution that carries us through.

ACKNOWLEDGMENTS

If you asked what I wanted to be when I grew up, I would've told you I longed to be an author. I have *always* loved stories.

Instead, I went to medical school and practiced medicine for nearly two decades and listened hard and cared for people and collected thousands and thousands of stories along the way. I once wrote an essay through tears about my patient in the NICU instead of catching up on sleep after a long night of call. Then I leaned back in my chair thinking, *Why did I write this?* Turns out, my passion for stories never went away.

This book, then, has truly been a team effort—a collection of stories from real women living good, hard, ordinary lives in what can sometimes be a wretched and miraculous world. It is my great privilege to have heard them and held them close and helped wherever I could and written them down and shared all these beautiful, heart-aching stories with other women. Our stories make the world go round, and today, I am thrilled to call myself an author.

Andy McGuire, thank you for believing in me. For listening and understanding and drawing me out and trusting the vision for this book. It is an honor to work with you. Thank you to everyone at Bethany House—the editing team and marketing group and publicity staff. You are all incredibly kind and encouraging and hardworking. And a special thank you to Her View From Home and its writers for supporting me along this writing path. I am so very grateful.

My beloved friends and *all* the women closest to me—Jenny and Angela and Amy and Emily and Mehr and Cassie and Diana and Angie and Michelle and Jenni and Amy and Amanda and Kari and Andrea and Rachel and Cherie—I couldn't imagine doing life without you. Thank you, thank you, thank you for putting up with me and loving me and swapping stories and forever being on my team.

Isaiah, Eli, James, Luke, and Lizzy, the five of you are *my favorite story of all time.* I love you. I love you like only a mom does. And I hope you'll always know it is my greatest gift to be your mom.

And Dan. Oh, how I love you. Thank you for walking alongside me, for carrying me whenever I am tired, and for holding my hand so tenderly along the way. Our life together as a family is truly my magnum opus.

APPENDIX 1

THE GAD-7 ANXIETY SCALE

* Score: 5 to 9 = mild anxiety; 10 to 14 = moderate anxiety; 15 to 21 = severe anxiety.

This is a form that can be printed out and filled out by hand rather than a calculator that can be filled in online.

Name:		Date:			
Over the last 2 weeks, how often have you been bothered by the following problems?					
	Not at all	Several days	More than half the days	Nearly every day	Total score
1. Feeling nervous, anxious, or on edge	0	1	2	3	
2. Not being able to stop or control worrying	0	1	2	3	
3. Worrying too much about different things	0	1	2	3	
4. Trouble relaxing	0	1	2	3	
5. Being so restless that it is hard to sit still	0	1	2	3	
6. Becoming easily annoyed or irritable	0	1	2	3	
7. Feeling afraid as if something awful might happen	0	1	2	3	
	____ +	____ +	____ +	____ =	____
If you checked off any problems, how difficult have these problems made it for you to do your work, take care of things at home, or get along with other people? (Circle one)	Not difficult at all	Somewhat difficult	Very difficult	Extremely difficult	

Developed by Drs. Robert L Spitzer, Janet BW Williams, Kurt Kroenke, and colleagues, with an educational grant from Pfizer, Inc. No permission required to reproduce, translate, display or distribute. Published in: Spitzer RL, Kroenke K, Williams JB, Lowe B. A brief measure for assessing generalized anxiety disorder: the GAD-7. Arch Intern Med 2006; 166:1092.

Graphic 77755 Version 23.0

APPENDIX 2

THE DAILY RECORD OF SEVERITY OF SYMPTOMS FOR PMDD

Name:												
Each evening note the degree to which you experienced each of the problems listed below on correct calendar day: 1—NOT AT ALL, 2—MINIMAL, 3—MILD, 4—MODERATE, 5—SEVERE, 6—EXTREME.												
Note spotting by entering "S", note menses by entering "M"												
Enter day (Monday = "M", Thursday = "R", etc)	1	2	3	4	5	6	7	8	9	10	11	12
1. Felt depressed, sad, "down", or "blue" or felt hopeless; or felt worthless or guilty												
2. Felt anxious, tense, "keyed up" or "on edge"												
3. Had mood swings (ie, suddenly feeling sad or tearful) or was sensitive to rejection or feelings were easily hurt												
4. Felt angry, or irritable												
5. Had less interest in usual activities (work, school, friends, hobbies)												
6. Had difficulty concentrating												
7. Felt lethargic, tired, or fatigued; or had lack of energy												
8. Had increased appetite or overate; or had cravings for specific foods												
9. Slept more, took naps, found it hard to get up when intended; or had trouble getting to sleep or staying asleep												
10. Felt overwhelmed or unable to cope; or felt out of control												
11. Had breast tenderness, breast swelling, bloated sensation, weight gain, headache, joint or muscle pain, or other physical symptoms												
At work, school, home, or in daily routine, at least one of the problems noted above caused reduction of productivity or inefficiency												
At least one of the problems noted above caused avoidance of or less participation in hobbies or social activities												
At least one of the problems noted above interfered with relationships with others												

Month/year:																		
13	14	15	16	17	18	19	20	21	22	23	24	25	26	27	28	29	30	31

THE PHQ-9 DEPRESSION QUESTIONNAIRE

Name:	Date:

Over the last 2 weeks, how often have you been bothered by any of the following problems?

	Not at all	Several days	More than half the days	Nearly every day	Total
Little interest or pleasure in doing things	0	1	2	3	
Feeling down, depressed, or hopeless	0	1	2	3	
Trouble falling or staying asleep, or sleeping too much	0	1	2	3	
Feeling tired or having little energy	0	1	2	3	
Poor appetite or overeating	0	1	2	3	
Feeling bad about yourself, or that you are a failure, or that you have let yourself or your family down	0	1	2	3	
Trouble concentrating on things, such as reading the newspaper or watching television	0	1	2	3	
Moving or speaking so slowly that other people could have noticed? Or the opposite, being so fidgety or restless that you have been moving around a lot more than usual.	0	1	2	3	
Thoughts that you would be better off dead, or of hurting yourself in some way	0	1	2	3	
	___	+ ___	+ ___	+ ___	___

PHQ-9 score ≥10: Likely major depression

Depression score ranges:

5 to 9: mild

10 to 14: moderate

15 to 19: moderately severe

≥20: severe

If you checked off any problems, how difficult have these problems made it for you to do your work, take care of things at home, or get along with other people? (Circle one)	Not difficult at all	Somewhat difficult	Very difficult	Extremely Difficult

Developed by Drs. Robert L Spitzer, Janet BW Williams, Kurt Kroenke, and colleagues, with an educational grant from Pfizer, Inc. No permission required to reproduce, translate, display or distribute.

Graphic 59307 Version 12.0

APPENDIX 4

SCREENING RECOMMENDATIONS FOR TRANSWOMEN AND TRANSMEN WITH PAST OR CURRENT HORMONE USE

	Transwomen (MTF)	Transmen (FTM)
Breast cancer	Discuss screening in patients >50 years with additional risk factors for breast cancer*	Intact breasts: Routine screening as for natal females
		Postmastectomy: Yearly chest wall and axillary exams¶
Cervical cancer	Vaginoplasty: No screening	Cervix intact: Routine screening as for natal females
		No cervix: No screening
Prostate cancer	Routine screening as for natal males	N/A
Cardiovascular disease	Screen for risk factors	Screen for risk factors
Diabetes mellitus	On estrogen: Increased risk	Routine screeningΔ
Hyperlipidemia	On estrogen: Annual lipid screening	On testosterone: Annual lipid screening
Osteoporosis	Testes intact: Routine screening as for natal males	Screen all patients >65 years Screen patients age 50 to 65 if off hormones for >5 years
	Postorchiectomy: Screen all patients >65 years Screen patients age 50 to 65 years if off hormones for >5 years	

* Estrogen/progestin therapy for >5 years, family history, body mass index (BMI) >35.

¶ While there is no evidence to support clinical breast examinations in this population, we perform yearly chest wall and axillary exams and use this as an opportunity to examine scar tissue, examine any changes, and educate the patient about the small but possible risk of breast cancer.

Δ Transmen with polycystic ovary syndrome (PCOS) should be screened for diabetes as for natal females with PCOS. Refer to the UpToDate material on further evaluation after diagnosis of PCOS in adults.

APPENDIX 5

TWO OPTIONS FOR HEALTHY EATING PLANS

The DASH Eating Plan

Daily Servings:

- Grains 6–8
- Meats, Poultry, and Fish 3–4 or fewer
- Vegetables 4–5
- Fruits 4
- Low-Fat Dairy Products 2–3
- Good Fats and Oils 2–3
- Sodium 2,300 mg (though a 1,500 mg daily diet will lower blood pressure more effectively)

Weekly Servings:

- Nuts, Seeds, and Beans 4–5
- Sweets 5 or less

***The DASH eating plan focuses on foods that are low in saturated and trans fats, rich in potassium, calcium, magnesium, fiber, and lean protein, and low in sodium.

The Mediterranean Eating Plan

Daily Servings:

- Grains and Starchy Vegetables 3–6
- Poultry and Eggs 1 or less of each

- Vegetables at least 3–5 or more
- Fruits 3
- Low-Fat Dairy Products 1 or less
- Extra Virgin Olive Oil 1–4
- Wine up to 1

Weekly Servings:

- Fish at least 3
- Nuts 3
- Red Meat 1 or less
- Sweets 3 or less

***The Mediterranean eating plan limits refined carbohydrates, sodium, sugar, and both saturated and trans fats while encouraging healthy omega-3 fatty acids and foods rich in fiber and antioxidants.

APPENDIX 6

REPUTABLE SITES FOR FURTHER READING

Centers for Disease Control and Prevention (CDC)
› CDC.gov

National Institutes of Health (NIH)
› NIH.gov/health-information

United States Preventative Services Task Force (USPSTF)
› USPreventiveServicesTaskForce.org/uspstf

National Library of Medicine (also called PubMed)
› PubMed.ncbi.nlm.nih.gov

North American Menopause Society (NAMS)
› Menopause.org

American College of Obstetricians and Gynecologists (ACOG)
› ACOG.org

National Center for Complementary and Integrative Health (NCCIH)
› NCCIH.nih.gov

Office of Research on Women's Health (ORWH)
› ORWH.od.nih.gov

NOTES

Introduction

1. This book could be a great resource for elite athletes who have reached middle age and want to maintain their peak physical performance. The book in your hands, however, is for the mostly ordinary rest of us who want to do the best we can to care for these bodies we *actually* have. Selene Yeager and Stacy T. Sims, PhD, *Next Level: Your Guide to Kicking Ass, Feeling Great, and Crushing Goals Through Menopause and Beyond* (Pennsylvania: Rodale, Inc, 2022).

Chapter 1 Promises of the "Beauty and Wellness" Industry

1. The already-massive beauty and wellness industry has grown to meet *endless* consumer demand. "The global wellness market is worth $4.4 trillion as of 2022. The U.S. wellness industry is valued at $1.2 trillion and makes up 28% of the worldwide wellness market as of 2021. The retail value of the U.S.'s health and wellness products is about $186 billion." Zippia. "28+ Enlightening Health and Wellness Industry Statistics [2023]: Facts, Data and Trends," Zippia.com, March 20, 2023, www.zippia.com/advice/health-and-wellness-industry-statistics.

2. "Normal." "Common." "Ideal." Merriam-Webster.com Dictionary, Merriam-Webster, www.merriam-webster.com/dictionary. Accessed 21 Jul. 2023.

3. According to the Centers for Disease Control National Center for Health Statistics, the average woman over 20 years of age in the US has the following measurements: "Height in inches: 63.5 Weight in pounds: 170.8 Waist circumference in inches: 38.7″ from www.cdc.gov/nchs/fastats/body-measurements.htm.

4. In medicine, we use both anecdotal and empirical evidence to generate hypotheses and then test them using randomized controlled trials. The results of such trials create evidence-based medical approaches and develop a gold standard for patient care. Arthur T. Evans, MD, MPH, and Gregory Mints, MD, FACP,

"Evidence-based Medicine," UpToDate, www.uptodate.com/contents/evidence
-based-medicine, accessed 23 Jul. 2023.

5. Henderson EL, Simons DJ, Barr DJ. The Trajectory of Truth: A Longitu-
dinal Study of the Illusory Truth Effect. J Cogn. 2021 Jun 8;4(1):29. https://doi
.org/10.5334/joc.161.

6. Our news feeds are full of misinformation. Let's learn how to be discerning.
Ioannidis JP. Why most published research findings are false. PLoS Med. 2005
Aug;2(8):e124. https://doi.org/10.1371/journal.pmed.0020124.

Chapter 2 So, *Could* It Be Your Thyroid???

1. "Nothing says responsible and OBVIOUSLY I'VE NEVER SPENT TIME
IN JAIL DON'T BE RIDICULOUS like a cardigan does." From the first of several
books I love from my favorite author. Glennon Doyle, *Carry On, Warrior: The
Power of Embracing Your Messy, Beautiful Life* (New York: Scribner, 2013), 151.

2. These are common vague symptoms in primary care and the differential
diagnosis of hypothyroidism. McDermott MT. Hypothyroidism. Ann Intern Med.
2020 Jul 7;173(1):ITC1-ITC16. https://doi.org/10.7326/AITC202007070.

3. Overview, incidence, symptoms of, and laboratory work for hypothyroidism. Wilson SA, Stem LA, Bruehlman RD. Hypothyroidism: Diagnosis and Treatment. Am Fam Physician. 2021 May 15;103(10):605–613. PMID: 33983002.

4. Primary vs. Secondary hypothyroidism definitions and evaluation for Hashimoto's thyroiditis. Ragusa F, Fallahi P, Elia G, Gonnella D, Paparo SR, Giusti C,
Churilov LP, Ferrari SM, Antonelli A. Hashimotos' thyroiditis: Epidemiology,
pathogenesis, clinic and therapy. Best Pract Res Clin Endocrinol Metab. 2019
Dec;33(6):101367. https://doi.org/10.1016/j.beem.2019.101367.

5. Treatment for hypothyroidism. Wilson SA, Stem LA, Bruehlman RD. Hypothyroidism: Diagnosis and Treatment. Am Fam Physician. 2021 May 15;103(10):
605–613. PMID: 33983002.

Chapter 3 Let's Talk about Stress

1. "Burnout is higher in sandwich generation caregivers and those who care
for parents than burnout among those who care only for children." Owsiany
MT, Fenstermacher EA, Edelstein BA. Burnout and Depression Among Sandwich Generation Caregivers: A Brief Report. Int J Aging Hum Dev. 2023 Jun
13:914150231183137. https://doi.org/10.1177/00914150231183137.

2. The autonomic nervous system—both the sympathetic and parasympathetic
systems—controls our body's response to stress through the amygdala and HPA
(hypothalamic-pituitary-adrenal) axis. Gibbons CH. Basics of autonomic nervous
system function. Handb Clin Neurol. 2019;160:407–418. https://doi.org/10.1016
/B978-0-444-64032-1.00027-8.

3. Our body's response is typically fight, flight, or freeze. Gibbons CH. Basics
of autonomic nervous system function. Handb Clin Neurol. 2019;160:407–418.
https://doi.org/10.1016/B978-0-444-64032-1.00027-8.

4. The fawn response helps us survive horrific events and may require extensive
therapy for recovery and repair. Pete Walker, *Complex PTSD: From Surviving to
Thriving* (An Azure Coyote Book, 2013), 13.

5. Pete Walker, *Complex PTSD*, 3.

6. The groundbreaking ACE study has now been expounded upon for decades as it relates to trauma-informed care. Felitti VJ, Anda RF, Nordenberg D, Williamson DF, Spitz AM, Edwards V, Koss MP, Marks JS. Relationship of childhood abuse and household dysfunction to many of the leading causes of death in adults. The Adverse Childhood Experiences (ACE) Study. Am J Prev Med. 1998 May; 14(4):245–58. https://doi.org/10.1016/s0749-3797(98)00017-8.

7. Chronic stress can be a risk factor for other chronic medical illnesses. Scott-Solomon E, Boehm E, Kuruvilla R. The sympathetic nervous system in development and disease. Nat Rev Neurosci. 2021 Nov;22(11):685-702. https://doi.org/10.1038/s41583-021-00523-y.

8. This book on stress for women should be a required reading. Emily Nagoski, PhD, and Amelia Nagoski, DMA, *Burnout: The Secret to Unlocking the Stress Cycle* (New York: Ballantine Books, 2020), 14–19.

9. Nagoski and Nagoski, *Burnout,* 15.

Chapter 4 How to Move Forward When Life Goes Completely off the Rails

1. Al-Anon and the "big blue book" radically changed my way of thinking and my tendency toward co-dependency. *How Al-Anon Works for Families & Friends of Alcoholics* (Al-Anon Family Groups, 1995).

2. This is my favorite daily prayer. *How Al-Anon Works for Families & Friends of Alcoholics*, 80.

3. Agency matters in our lives. Moore JW. What Is the Sense of Agency and Why Does It Matter? Front Psychol. 2016 Aug 29;7:1272. https://doi.org/10.3389/fpsyg.2016.01272.

4. Definition of limited agency. Moore JW. What Is the Sense of Agency and Why Does It Matter?

Chapter 5 "We Can Do Any(*EVERY*)thing" and Adult Attention Deficit Hyperactivity Disorder

1. To me, being a "feminist" means working toward *equal value*, not female superiority. It means respecting everyone's individual, informed choices and believing there shouldn't be a double standard. "Feminism" is about *all* humans having equal rights and opportunities, and it's about respecting every human being's diverse experience, identity, wisdom, and strength, empowering *all* humans to step fully into exactly who they've been created to be.

2. The authors of this book provide a new reason for inattention. Edward M. Hallowell, M.D., and John J. Ratey, M.D., *ADHD 2.0: New Science and Essential Strategies for Thriving with Distraction—from Childhood through Adulthood* (New York: Ballantine Books, 2022), 15.

3. "Cognitive load." APA Dictionary of Psychology, American Psychological Association, https://dictionary.apa.org/cognitive-load. Accessed 23 Jul. 2023.

4. An overview of adult ADHD. Salvi V, Migliarese G, Venturi V, Rossi F, Torriero S, Viganò V, Cerveri G, Mencacci C. ADHD in adults: clinical subtypes and associated characteristics. Riv Psichiatr. 2019 Mar-Apr;54(2):84–89. https://doi.org/10.1708/3142.31249.

5. Salvi, Migliarese, et al.. ADHD in adults.

6. Here's how we screen for ADHD. Anbarasan D, Kitchin M, Adler LA. Screening for Adult ADHD. Curr Psychiatry Rep. 2020 Oct 23;22(12):72. https://doi.org/10.1007/s11920-020-01194-9.

7. A self-report tool. Kessler RC, Adler L, Ames M, Demler O, Faraone S, Hiripi E, Howes MJ, Jin R, Secnik K, Spencer T, Ustun TB, Walters EE. The World Health Organization Adult ADHD Self-Report Scale (ASRS): a short screening scale for use in the general population. Psychol Med. 2005 Feb;35(2):245–56. https://doi.org/10.1017/s0033291704002892. Adapted for *UpToDate*, (UpToDate: Waltham, MA, 2023). Accessed 23 Jul. 2023.

8. American Psychiatric Association. *Diagnostic and Statistical Manual of Mental Disorders*, Fifth Edition, Text Revision (DSM-5-TR), Washington, DC, 2022.

9. Treatment combinations for ADHD. Caye A, Swanson JM, Coghill D, Rohde LA. Treatment strategies for ADHD: an evidence-based guide to select optimal treatment. Mol Psychiatry. 2019 Mar;24(3):390-408. https://doi.org/10.1038/s41380-018-0116-3.

10. This quote provides a perfect description of the ADHD brain. Thomas, Iain S., *I Wrote This For You: 2007–2017* (Missouri: Andrew McMeel Publishing, 2018).

Chapter 6 Rage, Premenstrual Dysphoric Disorder, and Changes of the Later Reproductive Years

1. Epidemiology statistics on PMS. Yonkers KA, Simoni MK. Premenstrual disorders. Am J Obstet Gynecol. 2018 Jan;218(1):68–74. https://doi.org/10.1016/j.ajog.2017.05.045.

2. Hantsoo L, Epperson CN. Premenstrual Dysphoric Disorder: Epidemiology and Treatment. Curr Psychiatry Rep. 2015 Nov;17(11):87. https://doi.org/10.1007/s11920-015-0628-3.

3. Here's an overview of the normal menstrual cycle. Schmalenberger KM, Tauseef HA, Barone JC, Owens SA, Lieberman L, Jarczok MN, Girdler SS, Kiesner J, Ditzen B, Eisenlohr-Moul TA. How to study the menstrual cycle: Practical tools and recommendations. Psychoneuroendocrinology. 2021 Jan;123:104895. https://doi.org/10.1016/j.psyneuen.2020.104895.

4. "The Menstrual Cycle," Encyclopedia Britannica, www.britannica.com/science/menstrual-cycle#/media/1/375292/112920.

5. Changes occur in the normal menstrual cycle during the later reproductive years. Allshouse A, Pavlovic J, Santoro N. Menstrual Cycle Hormone Changes Associated with Reproductive Aging and How They May Relate to Symptoms. Obstet Gynecol Clin North Am. 2018 Dec;45(4):613–628. https://doi.org/10.1016/j.ogc.2018.07.004.

6. Symptoms of PMDD. Bosman RC, Jung SE, Miloserdov K, Schoevers RA, Aan het Rot M. Daily symptom ratings for studying premenstrual dysphoric disorder: A review. J Affect Disord. 2016 Jan 1;189:43–53. https://doi.org/10.1016/j.jad.2015.08.063.

7. Endicott J, Nee J, Harrison W. Daily Record of Severity of Problems (DRSP): reliability and validity. Arch Womens Ment Health. 2006 Jan;9(1):41–9. https://doi.org/10.1007/s00737-005-0103-y.

8. Treatment of PMS and PMDD. Kenda M, Glavač NK, Nagy M, Sollner Dolenc M, On Behalf of the Oemonom. Herbal Products Used in Menopause and for Gynecological Disorders. Molecules. 2021 Dec 8;26(24):7421. https://doi.org/10.3390/molecules26247421.

9. SSRIs are commonly used for treatment of PMDD. Hantsoo L, Epperson CN. Premenstrual Dysphoric Disorder: Epidemiology and Treatment. Curr Psychiatry Rep. 2015 Nov;17(11):87. https://doi.org/10.1007/s11920-015-0628-3.

Chapter 7 What to Expect in Perimenopause

1. Symptoms of perimenopause. Santoro N, Roeca C, Peters BA, Neal-Perry G. The Menopause Transition: Signs, Symptoms, and Management Options. J Clin Endocrinol Metab. 2021 Jan 1;106(1):1-15. https://doi.org/10.1210/clinem/dgaa764.

2. Bacon JL. The Menopausal Transition. Obstet Gynecol Clin North Am. 2017 Jun;44(2):285–296. https://doi.org/10.1016/j.ogc.2017.02.008.

3. There are three main hormones that contribute to symptoms in perimenopause and the menopausal transition. Bacon JL. The Menopausal Transition.

4. This is an absolutely awesome book for all things menopause! Jen Gunter, MD, *The Menopause Manifesto: Own Your Health with Facts and Feminism* (New York: Kensington, 2021), 37.

5. Statistics for vasomotor symptoms during perimenopause. Avis NE, Crawford SL, Green R. Vasomotor Symptoms Across the Menopause Transition: Differences Among Women. Obstet Gynecol Clin North Am. 2018 Dec;45(4):629–640. https://doi.org/10.1016/j.ogc.2018.07.005.

6. Krause MS, Nakajima ST. Hormonal and nonhormonal treatment of vasomotor symptoms. Obstet Gynecol Clin North Am. 2015 Mar;42(1):163–79. https://doi.org/10.1016/j.ogc.2014.09.008.

7. Definitions of abnormal menstrual bleeding. Khafaga A, Goldstein SR. Abnormal Uterine Bleeding. Obstet Gynecol Clin North Am. 2019 Dec;46(4):595–605. https://doi.org/10.1016/j.ogc.2019.07.001.

8. Treatments for abnormal bleeding. Khafaga A, Goldstein SR. Abnormal Uterine Bleeding.

9. Here's how we evaluate postmenopausal bleeding. Carugno J. Clinical management of vaginal bleeding in postmenopausal women. Climacteric. 2020 Aug;23(4):343–349. https://doi.org/10.1080/13697137.2020.1739642.

10. Definition of metabolic syndrome and factors required for diagnosis. Bovolini A, Garcia J, Andrade MA, Duarte JA. Metabolic Syndrome Pathophysiology and Predisposing Factors. Int J Sports Med. 2021 Mar;42(3):199–214. https://doi.org/10.1055/a-1263-0898.

11. The menopausal transition can be associated with depression. Bromberger JT, Epperson CN. Depression During and After the Perimenopause: Impact of Hormones, Genetics, and Environmental Determinants of Disease. Obstet

Gynecol Clin North Am. 2018 Dec;45(4):663–678. https://doi.org/10.1016/j.ogc
.2018.07.007.

12. The SWAN study. El Khoudary SR, Greendale G, Crawford SL, Avis NE, Brooks MM, Thurston RC, Karvonen-Gutierrez C, Waetjen LE, Matthews K. The menopause transition and women's health at midlife: a progress report from the Study of Women's Health Across the Nation (SWAN). Menopause. 2019 Oct;26(10):1213–1227. https://doi.org/10.1097/GME.0000000000001424.

13. A discussion of menopausal hormone therapy. Troìa L, Martone S, Morgante G, Luisi S. Management of perimenopause disorders: hormonal treatment. Gynecol Endocrinol. 2021 Mar;37(3):195–200. https://doi.org/10.1080/09513590
.2020.1852544.

14. Some women cannot take MHT. Here's a look at risks and benefits. Rajan S, Kreatsoulas C. A review of menopausal hormone therapy: recalibrating the balance of benefit and risk. Pol Arch Intern Med. 2019 Apr 30;129(4):276–280. https://doi.org/10.20452/pamw.4412.

15. Menopause supplements. De Franciscis P, Colacurci N, Riemma G, Conte A, Pittana E, Guida M, Schiattarella A. A Nutraceutical Approach to Menopausal Complaints. Medicina (Kaunas). 2019 Aug 28;55(9):544. https://doi.org/10.3390
/medicina55090544.

16. Sood R, Shuster L, Smith R, Vincent A, Jatoi A. Counseling postmenopausal women about bioidentical hormones: ten discussion points for practicing physicians. J Am Board Fam Med. 2011 Mar–Apr;24(2):202–10. https://doi.org
/10.3122/jabfm.2011.02.100194.

17. Dietary Supplement Health and Education Act of 1994, Public Law 103-417, National Institutes of Health, https://ods.od.nih.gov/About/DSHEA_Word
ing.aspx.

Chapter 8 Loving the Body You *Actually* Have

1. Definitions of common eating disorders. American Psychiatric Association. *Diagnostic and Statistical Manual of Mental Disorders*, Fifth Edition, Text Revision (DSM-5-TR), Washington, DC, 2022, 271–277, 381–396.

2. Epidemiology and statistics of common eating disorders. Galmiche M, Déchelotte P, Lambert G, Tavolacci MP. Prevalence of eating disorders over the 2000–2018 period: a systematic literature review. Am J Clin Nutr. 2019 May 1;109(5):1402–1413. https://doi.org/10.1093/ajcn/nqy342.

3. This book is lifegiving. Hillary L. McBride, PhD, *The Wisdom of Your Body: Finding Healing, Wholeness, and Connection Through Embodied Living* (Grand Rapids, MI: Brazos Press, 2021), 87.

4. Samuels KL, Maine MM, Tantillo M. Disordered Eating, Eating Disorders, and Body Image in Midlife and Older Women. Curr Psychiatry Rep. 2019 Jul 1;21(8):70. https://doi.org/10.1007/s11920-019-1057-5.

5. Elise Loehnen, *On Our Best Behavior: The Seven Deadly Sins and the Price Women Pay to Be Good* (New York: The Dial Press, 2023), 131.

6. Our bodies have a set weight point when we stop yo-yo dieting. Rhee EJ. Weight Cycling and Its Cardiometabolic Impact. J Obes Metab Syndr. 2017 Dec 30;26(4):237–242. https://doi.org/10.7570/jomes.2017.26.4.237.

7. A must-see movie! *Barbie*, Greta Gerwig (California: Warner Bros, 2023).

8. Let's change our mindset about healthy eating and exercise. Gaesser GA, Angadi SS. Obesity treatment: Weight loss versus increasing fitness and physical activity for reducing health risks. iScience. 2021 Sep 20;24(10):102995. https://doi.org/10.1016/j.isci.2021.102995.

9. A great place to start for a mindset shift toward your body and appearance. Lindsay Kite, PhD, and Lexie Kite, PhD. *More Than a Body: Your Body Is an Instrument, Not an Ornament* (New York: Mariner Books, 2021), 290.

Chapter 9 Generalized Anxiety, Depression, and Other Mood Disorders

1. Definition of generalized anxiety. DeGeorge KC, Grover M, Streeter GS. Generalized Anxiety Disorder and Panic Disorder in Adults. Am Fam Physician. 2022 Aug;106(2):157–164. PMID: 35977134. https://pubmed.ncbi.nlm.nih.gov/35977134.

2. List of criteria for diagnosis of generalized anxiety. American Psychiatric Association. *Diagnostic and Statistical Manual of Mental Disorders*, Fifth Edition, Text Revision (DSM-5-TR), Washington, DC, 2022, 250–251.

3. Definition of depression. Trivedi MH. Major Depressive Disorder in Primary Care: Strategies for Identification. J Clin Psychiatry. 2020 Mar 17;81(2):UT-17042BR1C. https://doi.org/10.4088/JCP.UT17042BR1C.

4. List of criteria for diagnosis of depression. American Psychiatric Association. *Diagnostic and Statistical Manual of Mental Disorders*, Fifth Edition, Text Revision (DSM-5-TR), Washington, DC, 2022, 183.

5. Screening questionnaire for depression. Kroenke K, Spitzer RL, Williams JB. The Patient Health Questionnaire-2: validity of a two-item depression screener. Med Care. 2003 Nov;41(11):1284–92. https://doi.org/10.1097/01.MLR.0000093487.78664.3C.

6. Definition of dysthymia. Schramm E, Klein DN, Elsaesser M, Furukawa TA, Domschke K. Review of dysthymia and persistent depressive disorder: history, correlates, and clinical implications. Lancet Psychiatry. 2020 Sep;7(9):801–812. https://doi.org/10.1016/S2215-0366(20)30099-7.

7. Definition of seasonal affective disorder. Galima SV, Vogel SR, Kowalski AW. Seasonal Affective Disorder: Common Questions and Answers. Am Fam Physician. 2020 Dec 1;102(11):668–672. PMID: 33252911. https://pubmed.ncbi.nlm.nih.gov/33252911.

8. We use SSRIs for treatment of mood disorders. Edinoff AN, Akuly HA, Hanna TA, Ochoa CO, Patti SJ, Ghaffar YA, Kaye AD, Viswanath O, Urits I, Boyer AG, Cornett EM, Kaye AM. Selective Serotonin Reuptake Inhibitors and Adverse Effects: A Narrative Review. Neurol Int. 2021 Aug 5;13(3):387–401. https://doi.org/10.3390/neurolint13030038.

9. Psychotherapy is paramount for treatment of mood disorders. Cuijpers P, Quero S, Dowrick C, Arroll B. Psychological Treatment of Depression in Primary Care: Recent Developments. Curr Psychiatry Rep. 2019 Nov 23;21(12):129. https://doi.org/10.1007/s11920-019-1117-x.

10. Kristin Neff, PhD, *Self-Compassion: The Proven Power of Being Kind to Yourself* (New York: William Morrow, 2011), 12.

Chapter 10 Sex and Sleep: Bringing Sexy Back in Your (continuous positive airway pressure) CPAP Machine

1. A quote from my dear friend and fellow writer, Amy Betters-Midtvedt (@ amy.betters.midtvedt), "There was a time . . ." Instagram, October 24, 2021, www .instagram.com/p/CVbuigQrsKd.

2. Definition, diagnosis, and treatment of sleep apnea. Patel SR. Obstructive Sleep Apnea. Ann Intern Med. 2019 Dec 3;171(11):ITC81-ITC96. https://doi.org /10.7326/AITC201912030.

3. Statistics for sleep problems in women during midlife. Proserpio P, Marra S, Campana C, Agostoni EC, Palagini L, Nobili L, Nappi RE. Insomnia and menopause: a narrative review on mechanisms and treatments. Climacteric. 2020 Dec;23(6):539–549. https://doi.org/10.1080/13697137.2020.1799973.

4. Most sleep-aid medications have side effects. De Crescenzo F, D'Alò GL, Ostinelli EG, Ciabattini M, Di Franco V, Watanabe N, Kurtulmus A, Tomlinson A, Mitrova Z, Foti F, Del Giovane C, Quested DJ, Cowen PJ, Barbui C, Amato L, Efthimiou O, Cipriani A. Comparative effects of pharmacological interventions for the acute and long-term management of insomnia disorder in adults: a systematic review and network meta-analysis. Lancet. 2022 Jul 16;400(10347):170–184. https://doi.org/10.1016/S0140-6736(22)00878-9.

5. The average time for a woman to reach orgasm is 13 minutes. Bhat GS, Shastry A. Time to Orgasm in Women in a Monogamous Stable Heterosexual Relationship. J Sex Med. 2020 Apr;17(4):749–760. https://doi.org/10.1016/j.jsxm .2020.01.005.

6. Definition of genitourinary symptoms of menopause. Shifren JL. Genitourinary Syndrome of Menopause. Clin Obstet Gynecol. 2018 Sep;61(3):508–516. https://doi.org/10.1097/GRF.0000000000000380.

7. Definition of sexual interest/arousal disorder. Witherow-Párkányi M. Female sexual interest/arousal disorder: history of diagnostic considerations and their implications for clinical practice. Psychiatr Hung. 2022;37(2):133–149. https:// pubmed.ncbi.nlm.nih.gov/35582867.

8. Here are proven tactics to improve sleep. Baranwal N, Yu PK, Siegel NS. Sleep physiology, pathophysiology, and sleep hygiene. Prog Cardiovasc Dis. 2023 Mar–Apr;77:59–69. doi.org/10.1016/j.pcad.2023.02.005.

9. Treatment of genitourinary symptoms of menopause. Kagan R, Kellogg-Spadt S, Parish SJ. Practical Treatment Considerations in the Management of Genitourinary Syndrome of Menopause. Drugs Aging. 2019 Oct;36(10):897–908. https://doi.org/10.1007/s40266-019-00700-w.

Chapter 11 Dietary and "Natural" Supplements

1. Definition of non-GMO. Ambwani S, Sellinger G, Rose KL, Richmond TK, Sonneville KR. "It's Healthy Because It's Natural." Perceptions of "Clean" Eating among U.S. Adolescents and Emerging Adults. Nutrients. 2020 Jun 7;12(6):1708. https://doi.org/10.3390/nu12061708.

2. Bailey RL. Current regulatory guidelines and resources to support research of dietary supplements in the United States. Crit Rev Food Sci Nutr. 2020;60(2):298–309. https://doi.org/10.1080/10408398.2018.1524364.

3. Omega-3 supplementation has proven benefit. Watanabe Y, Tatsuno I. Prevention of Cardiovascular Events with Omega-3 Polyunsaturated Fatty Acids and the Mechanism Involved. J Atheroscler Thromb. 2020 Mar 1;27(3):183–198. https://doi.org/10.5551/jat.50658.

4. There are three parts to improving bone density: diet, activity, and supplementation. Rondanelli M, Faliva MA, Barrile GC, Cavioni A, Mansueto F, Mazzola G, Oberto L, Patelli Z, Pirola M, Tartara A, Riva A, Petrangolini G, Peroni G. Nutrition, Physical Activity, and Dietary Supplementation to Prevent Bone Mineral Density Loss: A Food Pyramid. Nutrients. 2021 Dec 24;14(1):74. https://doi.org/10.3390/nu14010074.

5. You only need to supplement if you don't get enough vitamin D in your diet. Rizzoli R. Vitamin D supplementation: upper limit for safety revisited? Aging Clin Exp Res. 2021 Jan;33(1):19–24. https://doi.org/10.1007/s40520-020-01678-x.

6. Fiber improves your health. Barber TM, Kabisch S, Pfeiffer AFH, Weickert MO. The Health Benefits of Dietary Fiber. Nutrients. 2020 Oct 21;12(10):3209. https://doi.org/10.3390/nu12103209.

Chapter 12 Preventive Care for Women in Midlife

1. Three Levels of Prevention, Merck Manual Consumer version, www.merckmanuals.com/home/multimedia/table/three-levels-of-prevention.

2. Cardiovascular disease prevention focuses on several aspects: blood pressure, blood sugars, cholesterol, smoking, and activity level. Arnett DK, Blumenthal RS, Albert MA, Buroker AB, Goldberger ZD, Hahn EJ, Himmelfarb CD, Khera A, Lloyd-Jones D, McEvoy JW, Michos ED, Miedema MD, Muñoz D, Smith SC Jr, Virani SS, Williams KA Sr, Yeboah J, Ziaeian B. 2019 ACC/AHA Guideline on the Primary Prevention of Cardiovascular Disease: A Report of the American College of Cardiology/American Heart Association Task Force on Clinical Practice Guidelines. Circulation. 2019 Sep 10;140(11):e596-e646. https://doi.org/10.1161/CIR.0000000000000678.

3. Breast cancer screening. Michaels E, Worthington RO, Rusiecki J. Breast Cancer: Risk Assessment, Screening, and Primary Prevention. Med Clin North Am. 2023 Mar;107(2):271–284. https://doi.org/10.1016/j.mcna.2022.10.007.

4. Smith RA, Andrews KS, Brooks D, Fedewa SA, Manassaram-Baptiste D, Saslow D, Wender RC. Cancer screening in the United States, 2019: A review of current American Cancer Society guidelines and current issues in cancer screening. CA Cancer J Clin. 2019 May;69(3):184–210. https://doi.org/10.3322/caac.21557.

5. Age of screening depends on underlying risk of breast cancer. US Preventive Services Task Force; Owens DK, Davidson KW, Krist AH, Barry MJ, Cabana M, Caughey AB, Doubeni CA, Epling JW Jr, Kubik M, Landefeld CS, Mangione CM, Pbert L, Silverstein M, Simon MA, Tseng CW, Wong JB. Risk Assessment, Genetic Counseling, and Genetic Testing for BRCA-Related Cancer: US Preventive Services Task Force Recommendation Statement. JAMA. 2019 Aug 20;322(7):652–665. https://doi.org/10.1001/jama.2019.10987.

6. Trajanoska K, Schoufour JD, de Jonge EAL, Kieboom BCT, Mulder M, Stricker BH, Voortman T, Uitterlinden AG, Oei EHG, Ikram MA, Zillikens MC, Rivadeneira F, Oei L. Fracture incidence and secular trends between 1989 and 2013

in a population based cohort: The Rotterdam Study. Bone. 2018 Sep;114:116–124. https://doi.org/10.1016/j.bone.2018.06.004.

7. Screening for osteoporosis. Viswanathan M, Reddy S, Berkman N, Cullen K, Middleton JC, Nicholson WK, Kahwati LC. Screening to Prevent Osteoporotic Fractures: Updated Evidence Report and Systematic Review for the US Preventive Services Task Force. JAMA. 2018 Jun 26;319(24):2532–2551. https://doi.org/10.1001/jama.2018.6537.

8. Leslie WD, Crandall CJ. Serial Bone Density Measurement for Osteoporosis Screening. JAMA. 2021 Oct 26;326(16):1622–1623. https://doi.org/10.1001/jama.2021.9858.

9. Screening for colon cancer. Bretthauer M, Løberg M, Wieszczy P, Kalager M, Emilsson L, Garborg K, Rupinski M, Dekker E, Spaander M, Bugajski M, Holme Ø, Zauber AG, Pilonis ND, Mroz A, Kuipers EJ, Shi J, Hernán MA, Adami HO, Regula J, Hoff G, Kaminski MF; NordICC Study Group. Effect of Colonoscopy Screening on Risks of Colorectal Cancer and Related Death. N Engl J Med. 2022 Oct 27;387(17):1547–1556. https://doi.org/10.1056/NEJMoa2208375.

10. Jain S, Maque J, Galoosian A, Osuna-Garcia A, May FP. Optimal Strategies for Colorectal Cancer Screening. Curr Treat Options Oncol. 2022 Apr;23(4):474–493. https://doi.org/10.1007/s11864-022-00962-4.

11. Stoffel EM, Murphy CC. Epidemiology and Mechanisms of the Increasing Incidence of Colon and Rectal Cancers in Young Adults. Gastroenterology. 2020 Jan;158(2):341–353. https://doi.org/10.1053/j.gastro.2019.07.055.

12. Cervical cancer statistics. Cohen PA, Jhingran A, Oaknin A, Denny L. Cervical cancer. Lancet. 2019 Jan 12;393(10167):169–182. https://doi.org/10.1016/S0140-6736(18)32470-X.

13. How we screen for cervical cancer. Bhatla N, Singhal S. Primary HPV screening for cervical cancer. Best Pract Res Clin Obstet Gynaecol. 2020 May;65:98–108. https://doi.org/10.1016/j.bpobgyn.2020.02.008.

14. Bhatla N, Singhal S. Primary HPV screening for cervical cancer.

15. The HPV vaccine for cervical cancer prevention. Athanasiou A, Bowden S, Paraskevaidi M, Fotopoulou C, Martin-Hirsch P, Paraskevaidis E, Kyrgiou M. HPV vaccination and cancer prevention. Best Pract Res Clin Obstet Gynaecol. 2020 May;65:109–124. https://doi.org/10.1016/j.bpobgyn.2020.02.009.

16. Here's a great tool for up-to-date screening recommendations: U.S. Preventative Services Task Force (USPSTF) A and B Recommendations. www.uspreventiveservicestaskforce.org/uspstf/recommendation-topics/uspstf-a-and-b-recommendations.

17. U.S. Preventative Services Task Force (USPSTF) A and B Recommendations.

18. Centers for Disease Control and Prevention (CDC), Immunization Schedule 2024, www.cdc.gov/vaccines/schedules/hcp/imz/adult.html#table-age, accessed March 6, 2024.

Chapter 13 Shame-based "Health" Practices vs. Love-based Healing

1. This book is an absolute must-read. Gabor Maté, MD, with Daniel Maté, *The Myth of Normal: Trauma, Illness, and Healing in a Toxic Culture* (New York: Avery, 2022), 20.

2. Hillary L. McBride, PhD, *The Wisdom of Your Body: Finding Healing, Wholeness, and Connection through Embodied Living* (Grand Rapids, MI: Brazos, 2021), 70.

Chapter 14 Seasons of Healing

1. Evaluating readiness for change. Krebs P, Norcross JC, Nicholson JM, Prochaska JO. Stages of change and psychotherapy outcomes: A review and meta-analysis. J Clin Psychol. 2018 Nov;74(11):1964–1979. https://doi.org/10.1002/jclp.22683.

2. The concept of small yesses for big wins. Britt Frank, MSW, LSCSW, Harness the Power of Your "Micro-Yes": Cracking the Procrastination Code. Psychology Today, February 18, 2023, www.psychologytoday.com/us/blog/the-science-of-stuck/202302/harness-the-power-of-your-micro-yes.

Chapter 15 Building a Team

1. Social connection is vital to our health. Holt-Lunstad J. Loneliness and Social Isolation as Risk Factors: The Power of Social Connection in Prevention. Am J Lifestyle Med. 2021 May 6;15(5):567–573. https://doi.org/10.1177/15598276211009454.

2. Ram Dass and Mirabai Bush, *Walking Each Other Home* (Boulder, CO: Sounds True, 2018).

INDEX

MIKALA ALBERTSON, MD

Dr. Mikala Albertson is a board-certified family practice doctor, author, and well-being advocate who is passionate about women's health and healing in the bodies we *actually* have in the lives we're *actually* living.

You'll find her most days in jeans and a T-shirt at the neighborhood grocery store stocking up on food for her teenagers, or at home attempting to keep laundry from overtaking the house. She loves hiking in the mountains, reading everything she can get her hands on, and writing *all* the words. But her main hobbies include picking up dirty socks and driving her kids from basketball practice to soccer games and back again.

More than anything, Mikala loves to tell the truth. She's the author of the book *Ordinary on Purpose: Surrendering Perfect and Discovering Beauty amid the Rubble*. And she encourages readers daily to lay down the chase for a "perfect" life or some unattainable cultural ideal of "beauty and wellness" and, instead, aim for wholehearted living using a more gentle, achievable, and sustainable approach. Her greatest hope for writing is to give you permission to live fully in a life that is *yours*.

Mikala and her relentlessly kind and patient husband are raising their five amazing children near Salt Lake City, Utah.

Connect with Mikala Albertson:
MikalaAlbertsonMD.com
Facebook [@MikalaAlbertsonMD]
Instagram [@MikalaAlbertsonMD]